Study Guide for the

NATA

BOARD OF CERTIFICATION, INC.

Entry-Level
Athletic Trainer

CERTIFICATION EXAMINATION

Study Guide for the

NATA

BOARD OF CERTIFICATION, INC.

Entry-Level Athletic Trainer

CERTIFICATION EXAMINATION

THIRD EDITION

Douglas M. Kleiner, PhD, ATC, CSCS, EMT, FACSM
Associate Professor

University of North Florida
Jacksonville, Florida

University of Florida
Health Science Center—Jacksonville
Jacksonville, Florida

F. A. DAVIS COMPANY / PUBLISHERS • PHILADELPHIA

F. A. Davis Company
1915 Arch Street
Philadelphia, PA 19103
www.fadavis.com

Printed in the United States of America

ISBN 0-8036-0785-7

Last digit indicates print number: 10 9 8 7 6 5 4 3 2 1

Acquisitions Editor: Christa A. Fratantoro
Production Editor: Jessica Howie Martin
Cover Designer: Louis J. Forgione

This study guide is dedicated to my mother and the memory of my father. They, along with my brothers and sister, encouraged me and showed me, by example, how to become a success.

Foreword

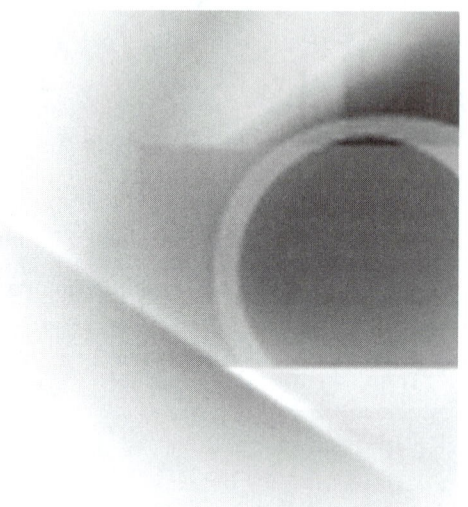

The fact that you are reading this study guide indicates that you have completed, or are nearing completion of, your athletic training education. Although the National Athletic Trainers' Association Board of Certification (NATABOC) examination for entry-level athletic trainers may seem a hurdle, it is, in fact, a gateway for entry into the profession.

The purpose of the NATABOC examination process is to ensure that certified athletic trainers demonstrate the knowledge and skill required to practice our profession safely, thereby benefitting athletes and the public. Also, the ATC certificate is a prerequisite for obtaining licensure in most states. Thus, by passing the certification examination, you are passing through the gateway into professional practice.

This study guide is a tool to guide you through your preparation for the certification examination. It is NOT intended to provide you with the cognitive knowledge or psychomotor skills necessary to pass the examination. You have gained this knowledge and these skills in your formal coursework and clinical education. Now, with this study guide, you can refine that knowledge and understand how the written, simulation, and practical sections of the NATABOC examination are administered.

The inclusion of domain-specific practice questions in the chapter on the written examination will help you to identify your areas of strength and weakness. After taking the test and calculating your score per domain, concentrate on studying your old class notes, textbooks, and other references to refresh your knowledge in these domains. You can then refer back to the domain-specific practice questions to continue to improve your scores.

The enclosed CD-ROM generates a random assortment of test questions that closely reflect the type of questions that you will actually face on the certification examination. To concentrate on a particular domain, you may select questions from that domain.

Although most of your focus will be on the areas in which you did poorly, do not neglect the areas in which you scored better. The post-test can serve as an indicator of your progress in obtaining your ultimate goal: becoming a certified athletic trainer.

Almost as important as studying is understanding the test day procedures. Sitting for the examination for the first time can be an intimidating experience. Knowing what the testing environment is like and understanding the test expectations and process can help reduce your anxiety and improve your score.

Although the gateway may seem rather small, it is one that can easily be opened by using the right key—the key of professional competence.

CHAD STARKEY, PhD, ATC
Chair, NATA Education Council
Boston, Massachusetts

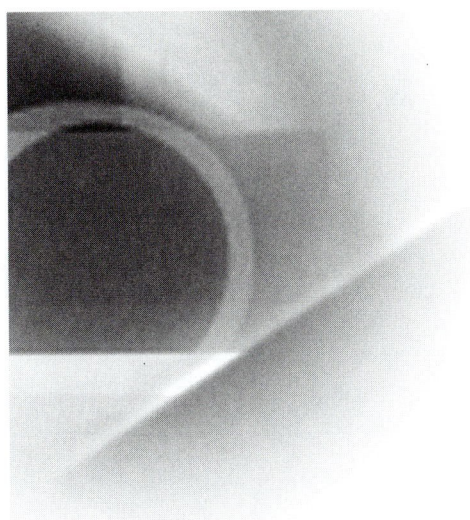

Preface

The role of this study guide, like that of most study guides, is not to augment a candidate's educational preparation, but to give the candidate useful information on how the examination is developed and scored and to provide a sample of the types of questions that could be asked on the certification examination.

To use this guide effectively, candidates should pay special attention to the information provided about each portion of the examination. Most candidates are experienced in taking multiple-choice examinations. However, many have limited experience with practical and simulation-type tests. Every effort should be made to be very deliberate when reviewing information about the practical and simulation portions of the examination. The sample simulation questions in this study guide provide an excellent example of the types and structure of the questions that are on the actual examination. This is the only study guide for the athletic training certification examination to provide the same latent-image format used on the National Athletic Trainers' Association Board of Certification (NATABOC) examination.

Neither the author nor F. A. Davis makes any claims about how successful a candidate using this guide will or will not be on the NATABOC certification examination. To expect one small book to contain the body of knowledge necessary for this profession is unthinkable. However, when used for its intended purpose, this guide can provide valuable assistance to candidates in preparing for the test. I wish you good luck in your preparation and much success on the examination.

DOUGLAS M. KLEINER

Acknowledgments

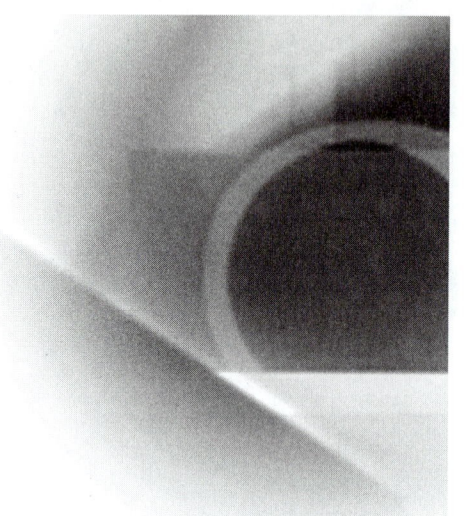

I would like to thank all the individuals who contributed to this revision, including many of my former students at Illinois State University and at the University of North Florida. Thanks as well to Denise Fandell for all her help.

I would also like to thank all my teachers, mentors, and colleagues who taught me so much throughout the years.

I especially want to thank Denny Aten, Rob Doyle, and Cheryl Birkhead at Eastern Illinois University for their contributions, and Chad Starkey, Joe Beckett, Kim Terrell, Charlie Hardaker, and David Pearson for their reviews.

Finally, a special note of thanks goes to Chad Starkey for being a friend and for writing the foreword to this guide.

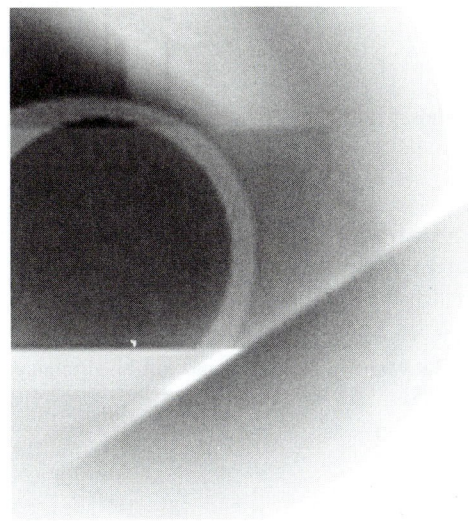

Contents

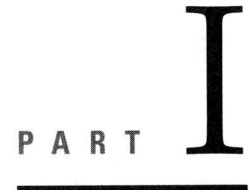

PART I

The Content and Process for the NATABOC Certification Examination

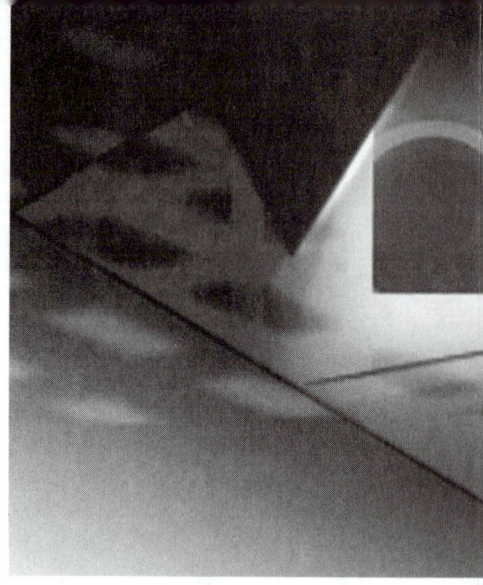

CHAPTER 1

Eligibility for the Examination

To be eligible to sit for the National Athletic Trainers Association Board of Certification (NATABOC) athletic training certification examination, candidates must meet a number of academic and clinical requirements. Currently, there are two ways to meet these standards: through an accredited athletic training education program and through an internship. However, internship will be discontinued as an avenue for athletic trainer certification examination eligibility on January 1, 2004.

At some point during your education, your supervising athletic trainer or athletic training program director should have familiarized you with the NATABOC Role Delineation Study (Chap. 4) and the NATABOC Standards for Athletic Training (Appendix A). If you are not familiar with these, please take the time now to familiarize yourself with these important documents.

Candidates may sit for the certification examination during their last quarter or semester on the test date closest to graduation, provided that all academic and clinical requirements have been met **at the time of application.** However, certification is not granted until candidates show proof of graduation.

◼ CURRICULUM CANDIDATES

Candidates in this category must successfully complete a program accredited by the Commission for the Accreditation of Allied Health Education Programs (CAAHEP) on recommendation by the Joint Review Committee on Athletic Training (JRC-AT). These programs have shown compliance with academic and clinical requirements meeting the NATABOC eligibility standards.

◼ INTERNSHIP CANDIDATES

Individuals who are not enrolled in programs accredited by CAAHEP are considered internship candidates. This is a practical education-work experience approach to certification eligibility.

NOTE: The National Athletic Trainers Association (NATA) and NATABOC are discontinuing internship as a way to certification examination eligibility. As of January 1, 2004, you must be a graduate of a CAAHEP-accredited athletic training education program in order to take the certification examination. To take the examination through the internship route, completed applications must be accepted by the NATABOC before December 31, 2003.

◼ APPLYING FOR THE EXAMINATION

To receive an internship application for the examination (Figure 1–1) or to receive more information regarding examination eligibility and fees, please contact

CASTLE Worldwide™, Inc.
120 First Flight Lane
Morrisville, NC 27560
(919) 572–6880, ext. 128
(fax) (919) 361–2426

Candidates from a CAAHEP-accredited athletic training education program must receive their curriculum candidate certification examination application (Figure 1–2) from their athletic training program director.

NAME (Please Print) _____
                                      Last   First   MI

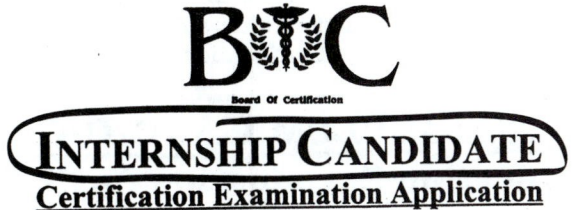

INSTRUCTIONS TO CANDIDATES

1. Applications must be **complete** at the time of application.
2. Your check must be made payable to NATABOC *or* complete credit card information submitted.
3. You may attach additional sheets as necessary. Complete information is required or your application will be returned to you.
4. Forward this application in the self-addressed envelope provided.

> **NATABOC**
> c/o Columbia Assessment Services, Inc.
> 120 First Flight Lane
> Morrisville, NC 27560

TEST DATE AND SITE SELECTION

Please refer to the enclosed Guidelines for Selecting Test Dates and the Exam Schedule before listing choices.
If you have not completed all of your required educational coursework you may still take the test, but **only** on the test date closest to your graduation. Indicate your test site selection(s) below.

Exam Date #1 _____ (My first choice test date)	**Exam Date #2** _____ (My second choice if Exam Date #1 is closed)
Site #1 _____	Site #1 _____
Site #2 _____	Site #2 _____
Site #3 _____	Site #3 _____
Site #4 _____	Site #4 _____
Site #5 _____	Site #5 _____
Site #6 _____	Site #6 _____
Site #7 _____	Site #7 _____

NOTE: If you require special testing accommodations, please complete the form that pertains to ADA testing accommodations, and enclose documentation of your disability along with a description of the type of testing arrangements you require.

The National Athletic Trainers Association Board of Certification, Inc. (NATABOC), does not discriminate against any individual on the basis of religion, gender, ethnic background, or physical disability.

NATABOC reserves the right to reject any application which does not meet application requirements.

Figure 1-1 Internship Candidate Certification Examination Application.

Name (Please Print):_____

| Last | First | MI |

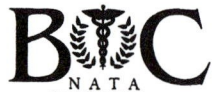

NATABOC, Inc.
National Athletic Trainers Association
Board of Certification, Inc.

CURRICULUM CANDIDATE
Certification Examination Application

The National Athletic Trainers Association Board of Certification, Inc. (NATABOC), does not discriminate against any individual on the basis of religion, gender, ethnic background, or physical disability.

NATABOC reserves the right to reject any application which does not meet application requirements.

When filling out the application: It is necessary to provide complete information as requested. You may attach additional sheets to the application, as needed. It is your responsibility to notify NATABOC of any changes in the information herein within 15 days prior to the examination.

When submitting the application: Please follow the enclosed Curriculum Candidate Checklist. All materials listed on the Checklist must be enclosed with this application. **Incomplete applications will not be approved.** Your check should be made payable to NATABOC. Applications received after the deadline will be returned.

Forward this application to the following address only:

If sending via regular U.S. Mail:

NATABOC, Inc.
P.O. Box 14148
Research Triangle Park, NC 27709-4148

> *If sending by Federal Express, UPS, or U.S. Certified or Express Mail, please mail to:*
>
> *NATABOC, Inc.*
> *120 First Flight Lane*
> *Morrisville, NC 27560*

TEST DATE AND SITE SELECTION

Please refer to the instructions on the back of the enclosed testing schedule before listing choices.

EXAM DATE #1 _____
(My first choice test date)
Site #1_____
Site #2_____
Site #3_____
Site #4_____
Site #5_____
Site #6_____

EXAM DATE #2 _____
(My second choice if Exam Date #1 is closed)
Site #1_____
Site #2_____
Site #3_____
Site #4_____
Site #5_____
Site #6_____

* *If you require special testing accommodations: Please complete the enclosed form that pertains to ADA testing accommodations, and enclose documentation of your disability along with the type of testing arrangements you require.*

Figure 1–2 Curriculum Candidate Certification Examination Application.

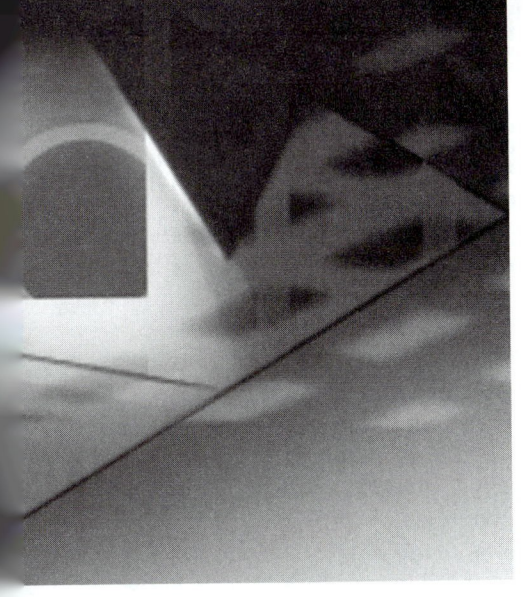

CHAPTER 2

Examination Information from the National Athletic Trainers Association Board of Certification

MISSION STATEMENT

The mission of the National Athletic Trainers Association Board of Certification (NATABOC) is to certify athletic trainers and to identify quality health care professionals for the public through a system of certification, adjudication, standards of practice, and continuing competency programs.

The NATABOC was incorporated in 1989 to provide a certification program for entry-level athletic trainers and recertification standards for certified athletic trainers (ATCs). An eight-member Board of Directors, consisting of five athletic trainer directors, one physician director, one public director, and one corporate/educational director, governs the NATABOC.

The NATABOC is the only accredited certification program for athletic trainers in the United States. Every 5 years the NATABOC must undergo review and reaccreditation by the National Commission for Certifying Agencies (NCCA). The NCCA is the accreditation body of the National Organization for Competency Assurance (NOCA).

Purpose of Certification

The purpose of this entry-level certification program is to establish standards for entry into the profession of athletic training. In addition, the NATABOC has established the continuing education requirements necessary to maintain status as an NATABOC-certified athletic trainer.

To Be Certified

In order to attain certification as an athletic trainer, a candidate must (1) satisfy the basic requirements, (2) satisfy the section requirements used to meet eligibility requirements, and (3) pass a three-part national certification examination.

The Process

Annually, the Board of Certification reviews the requirements for certification eligibility and standards for continuing education. In addition, the Board reviews and revises the certification examination in accordance with the test specifications of the NATABOC Role Delineation Study, which is reviewed and revised every 5 years. The Board of Certification uses a criterion-referenced passing point for the anchor form of the examination. Each new examination version is equated with the anchor version to ensure that candidates are not rewarded or penalized for taking different versions of the examination.

▇ REQUIREMENTS FOR CANDIDACY

A. Basic Requirements

Please note: If any of the basic requirements are not fulfilled at the time of application, the application will be returned to the applicant. There are no exceptions.

1. The athletic training student must have a high school diploma to begin accumulating the supervised athletic training experience hours that are to be used to meet requirements for NATABOC certification.

2. Candidates must supply proof of graduation (an official transcript) at the baccalaureate level from an accredited college or university located in the United States of America. Graduates of foreign universities may petition for a substitution of this degree requirement. Such a request will be evaluated at the candidate's expense by an independent consultant selected by the NATABOC.

    Students who have enrolled in their last semester or last quarter of college may apply to take the certification examination before graduation provided that all academic and clinical requirements of the section used for candidacy have been satisfied. A candidate will be permitted to take the examination on the date closest to his or her date of graduation.

Any internship applicant applying to take the examination before graduation must submit written verification of intent to graduate from the dean or department chairperson of the college or university from which the applicant will graduate. Applicants who have not completely satisfied the academic course requirements must submit a letter from the college registrar verifying enrollment in the required class(es). Certification will not be issued until the Board of Certification receives an official transcript indicating successful completion of all athletic training coursework and the date of degree. Course requirements for the internship route are shown in Table 2–1.

3. Candidates must supply proof of current certification in cardiopulmonary resuscitation (CPR) (course must include adult CPR techniques) from one of the following acceptable providers: American Red Cross, American Heart Association, National Safety Council, or EMP America. A photocopy of a valid CPR card or proof of enrollment in a course must be attached to the application. Current emergency medical technician (EMT) certification is an acceptable alternative for satisfying the CPR requirement. CPR certification must be current at the time of application.

4. At the time of application, a candidate for certification must verify that at least 25 percent (200 hours for accredited curriculum or 375 hours for internship applicants) of the required athletic training experience hours credited in fulfilling the certification requirements were obtained in actual (on location) practice and or game coverage with one or more of the following sports: football, soccer, hockey, wrestling, basketball, gymnastics, lacrosse, volleyball, rugby, and rodeo.

5. The certification application must be endorsed by an NATABOC-certified athletic trainer.

TABLE 2–1	COURSE REQUIREMENTS FOR CANDIDATES APPLYING THROUGH THE INTERNSHIP ROUTE

Health (i.e., nutrition, drugs/substance abuse, health education, pathology, personal health)
Human anatomy
Kinesiology/biomechanics
Human physiology
Physiology of exercise
Basic athletic training
Advanced athletic training*

*The **only** acceptable alternative for advanced athletic training is one course in therapeutic modalities **and** one course in rehabilitative exercise.

B. Section Requirements

1. Section One: Graduate of an entry-level curriculum accredited by the Commission for the Accreditation of Allied Health Education Programs (CAAHEP)

    Candidates from this section must successfully complete an entry-level athletic training program accredited by CAAHEP in no less than 2 academic years. The NATABOC will not accept athletic training hours that were accumulated more than 5 years before the application date. The program must include 800 hours of athletic training experience under the supervision of an NATABOC-certified athletic trainer. The athletic training experiences must be obtained from athletic training settings associated with the accredited curriculum.

2. Section Two: Internship

    At the time of application, each internship applicant must present documentation of at least 1500 hours of athletic training experience under the supervision of an NATABOC-certified athletic trainer. The applicant must show proof that the athletic training experience was gained over a period of at least 2 academic years. The NATABOC will not accept athletic training hours that were accumulated more than 5 years before the application date. Of these 1500 hours, at least 1000 hours must be attained in a traditional athletic training setting at the interscholastic, intercollegiate, or professional sports level. The additional 500 hours may be attained from an allied clinical setting or sport camp setting, or both, under the supervision of an NATABOC-certified athletic trainer. All athletic training experience hours must be completed at the time of application. Applicants applying for candidacy must submit an official transcript that verifies successful completion of the course requirements as indicated in Table 2–1.

    Beginning January 1, 2001, Basic and Advanced Athletic Training classes incorporated content in the following areas: prevention of athletic injuries, recognition and management of acute athletic injuries, rehabilitation of athletic injuries, therapeutic modalities, and evaluation of injury.

    Although not required, the NATABOC strongly recommends that candidates also receive instruction in the following content areas: physics, pharmacology, health care administration, professional development and responsibility, recognition of medical conditions, chemistry, psychosocial intervention and referral, nutrition, and pathology of injury and illness.

▥ DEFINITION OF TERMS

The following definitions are applicable to all potential candidates for certification by the NATABOC. These definitions should be used as a guideline and reference throughout the certification process. For additional terms, see Appendix B.

A. Endorsing Certified Athletic Trainer

1. *For the internship applicant*, this person is the NATABOC-certified athletic trainer who endorses the internship applicant's application for certification and who supervises at least 33 percent of the 1500 athletic training experience hours required under this section.

2. *For the accredited curriculum applicant*, this person is the NATABOC-certified athletic trainer or person with equivalent qualifications who endorses a curriculum graduate's application for certification. This person must be identified as the athletic training program director at the applicant's college or university by the accrediting agency. If the endorsing ATC withdraws his or her endorsement, the NATABOC may suspend the application. The candidate will be notified if the endorsement of his or her application has been withdrawn and will be advised of the consequences of this action.

B. Athletic Trainer Certified (ATC) or Certified Athletic Trainer (CAT)

    An athletic trainer certified or a certified athletic trainer is an allied health professional with a bachelor's degree from an accredited college or university who has fulfilled the requirements for certification as established by the NATABOC and has passed the certification examination administered by the NATABOC.

C. Athletic Training Student

    An athletic training student is an individual who is fulfilling the requirements for certification.

D. Athletic Training Setting for Acceptable Athletic Training Experience

1. *Primary Setting:* The primary setting is the athletic training facility that serves as the physical setting at which the minimum hours of direct supervision are accumulated.

    Athletic training facility is defined as "a designated physical facility located within an educational institution or professional sports complex in which comprehensive health care services are provided to competitive athletes." The athletic training facility must provide at least the following equipment: taping table(s), treatment table(s), heat and cold therapy (e.g., ice, hydrocollator, whirlpool), emergency equipment (e.g., splints, crutches, stretcher), first aid supplies, therapeutic exercise equipment (e.g., hand and leg weights, surgical tubing), and a record-keeping system (e.g., file cabinet, injury record forms). Comprehensive athletic health care services include, but are not limited to, prepractice and pregame preparation (taping, bandaging, application of protective padding, etc.), injury and illness evaluation; first-aid and emergency care, follow-up rehabilitation, and related services.

2. *Secondary Setting:* The secondary setting may include athletic practice and game coverage (home and away) and on-campus satellite athletic training rooms.

3. *Allied Setting:* The allied setting may include sports medicine clinics, summer sports camps, sports performance facilities, and varied hospital facilities.

E. Unacceptable Athletic Training Experience Hours and Coursework

1. Hours not spent under the supervision of an ATC

2. Hours spent traveling (team travel, lodging, etc.)

3. Hours earned more than 5 academic years before the date of the application for the certification examination

4. A course that does not satisfy the definition of a formal course (i.e., a workshop or practicum), a course in which the applicant received a failing grade, an audited course

F. Supervision

1. Supervision involves daily personal or verbal contact, or both, at the site of supervision between the athletic training student and the ATC who plans, directs, advises, and evaluates the student's athletic training experience. The supervising ATC must be physically present in order to intervene on behalf of the individual being treated. Hours that are not supervised by an ATC will not count toward certification requirements.

2. For internship applicants, all athletic training experiences that are to be credited toward satisfying the athletic training experience (hours) requirement must be documented on Verification of Hours forms and submitted with the certification examination application. A form is required from each ATC who supervised hours.

3. Internship route applicants who are supervised by athletic trainers certified by the Canadian Athletic Therapists Association (CATA) may receive credit for up to one third (500 hours) of the athletic training experience (hours) requirement.

4. Supervision provided by ATCs under the following conditions **will not** be accepted by the NATABOC:
   a. Supervision of the employer of an ATC or other individual who can alter the athletic trainer's conditions of employment or employment status, or both
   b. Supervision of a relative, spouse, or domestic partner

G. Supervising Athletic Trainer

Certified athletic trainers who are supervising educational experiences of athletic training students shall afford supervision adequate to ensure (following stated written and verbal direction) that the student performs his or her tasks in a manner consistent with the Standards of Practice of the profession of Athletic Training. To satisfy the eligibility requirements, ATCs supervising athletic training students must be recognized as athletic trainers at the setting where athletic training experience hours are being obtained. Each ATC must maintain a record of each student's experiential hours for future reference by the NATABOC.

H. Basic Requirements

Basic requirements are defined as requirements that all applicants must fulfill before their applications will be accepted for candidacy granted by the NATABOC.

I. Graduate of an Accredited Curriculum

The applicant must be a graduate of an accredited entry-level program of study in athletic training education accredited by the CAAHEP. Graduates of these programs are referred to as curriculum graduates.

J. Internship Route to Candidacy

The internship route to certification is a practical/education/work experience approach to gaining the knowledge and skills needed to fulfill the requirements for certification. Learning opportunities are designed by a student and an ATC to satisfy the eligibility requirements for internship candidacy. Athletic training students of this type are referred to as interns. The NATABOC does not review, sanction, or endorse educational opportunities identified as "athletic training internship programs." These "programs" are independent of any formal review by the NATABOC.

K. Formal Course or Formal Coursework

A formal course or formal coursework involves instruction and the teaching of appropriate knowledge and skills as course content in a structured classroom environment in the required subject content area.

Each course within an athletic training curriculum must be assigned academic credit for it to be accepted by the Board of Certification. Practicum or internship-based courses may not be substituted for formal coursework. Internship applicants must include a copy of the course descriptions (from their college catalogue) and course syllabi for courses used to satisfy the academic course requirements. In addition, internship applicants must highlight on their transcript(s) the courses used to satisfy the academic requirements. **Applications received without highlighted transcripts, course descriptions, or course syllabi may be returned to the applicant and will not be processed.**

Continuing education credit courses are not acceptable for satisfying the academic course requirements for examination eligibility. Independent study courses may be used to satisfy an academic course requirement, although academic credit must be assigned to an independent study course. Failing grades or audits will not be accepted.

▦ GUIDELINES FOR SELECTING TEST DATES AND TEST SITES FOR NATABOC EXAMINATION

Space is limited at all NATABOC test sites. Therefore, seats are assigned objectively on a "first come, first served" basis. Depending on when the application arrives at the testing office, a candidate's desired test sites may or may not have openings. It is recommended that applications be forwarded **as early as possible** before the deadline date.

Instructions for Selecting Test Dates and Sites

Please refer to the bottom portion of the front page of your NATABOC application.

NOTE: **If you are a graduating college senior and are applying before graduation, you may take the examination only on the closest examination date before your graduation.**

1. Begin by listing your first-choice test date next to **Exam Date #1.** Then, underneath Exam Date #1, list all test sites where you can attend on your first-choice test date. Consider all cities listed on the examination schedule to which you can reasonably travel. **You may attach a separate sheet of paper listing additional sites for Exam Date #1, if needed.**

2. Next, list your second choice test date next to **Exam Date #2,** in case your choices for Exam Date #1 are closed. Under Exam Date #2, list **all** test sites where you could attend on your second-choice day. **You may attach a separate sheet of paper, if needed.**

The NATABOC will make every effort to seat you for the first available test site under your first-choice test date (Exam Date #1). However, if all the sites you select for your first-choice test date are filled, the NATABOC will automatically seat you for a site on your second-choice test date (Exam Date #2).

IMPORTANT NOTE

It is imperative that you list **all** test sites you can attend on your first-choice test date when you mail the application. Once your application arrives at the NATABOC office, you will **not** be able to choose additional sites. If all the sites you chose for Exam Date #1 are full and you are automatically seated for Exam Date #2, you will **not** be able to select alternates for Exam Date #1.

There are no "waiting lists" for test sites that have reached capacity.

If all the sites you selected for your first-choice test date are closed and you did **not** list a second-choice test date with sites, you cannot be seated and your application and payment will be returned to you by U.S. mail.

If you have any questions regarding registration and seat assignment, please feel free to contact the NATABOC Account Representative at 919–572–6880, ext. 128.

Application Information

1. Application forms should be requested at least 4 months before the examination date. On receipt of the form, the certification office will review the information and assess the applicant's eligibility to sit for the examination. Applicants are accepted and scheduled in order of receipt. Applications and information can be obtained from the NATABOC offices and also may be downloaded from the

NATABOC homepage at www.nataboc.org/Internship Application.

2. A 75-percent refund of the exam fee will be issued if cancellation is made in writing and received no later than the deadline date for the exam.
3. Fifty percent of the exam fee will be refunded if cancellation is made after the deadline date. This policy will also apply to "no shows."
4. The fee for rescheduling an examination is $100.
5. The certification examination is administered five times a year at various locations across the United States.

Confirmation of Scheduling

After receipt of your NATABOC Certification Examination application, the NATABOC testing company, CASTLE Worldwide, Inc. (formerly Columbia Assessment Services [CAS], Inc.), will provide you with written confirmation of your exam registration. This is sent via U.S. mail.

You will receive an admission ticket 2 to 3 weeks before the examination date. The exact time and location of the examination are printed on the ticket. Candidates must bring the ticket to the examination.

Cost of the Examination

	2001 Exam Fees
First-Time Candidate—Members	$300
First-Time Candidate—Nonmembers	$350
Retake: One Section	$190
Retake: Two Sections	$235
Retake: Three Sections	$275

All certification examination candidates must review the requirements for certification contained in the credentialing information brochure. The brochure is available on the NATABOC website.

To receive an internship application via U.S. mail, please contact the NATABOC at www.staff@nataboc.org. A curriculum application can be obtained by contacting the program director of the accredited athletic training program of attendance.

IMPORTANT NOTE

Completed applications must be **received by (not postmarked by)** the prescribed deadline date for the examination date chosen. Test sites often fill before the deadline date.

Mailing an application does not guarantee a seat at any test site.

EXAMINATION RULES

1. No books, papers, or other reference materials may be taken into the examination room. An area will be provided for the storage of such materials.
2. No examination materials, documents, or memoranda of any type are to be taken from the room.
3. The examination will be given only on the date and time noted on the admission ticket. If an emergency arises and you are unable to take the examination as scheduled, you should call CASTLE Worldwide, Inc. on the day of the examination.
4. No questions concerning the content of the examination may be asked during the examination period. You should listen carefully to the directions given by the proctor and read the directions carefully in the examination booklet.

POLICY FOR SPECIAL ACCOMMODATION: ACCOMMODATION PROCEDURES

1. An applicant may request a change in certification procedures or process because of a physical or learning disability or other reasons. A specific form, available from the NATABOC, must be completed and received by the NATABOC before the deadline of the requested examination date.
2. The request must be specific as to the nature of the problem. Medical documentation of specific needs must accompany the request. The applicant is responsible for demonstrating that the request should be granted. The Board of Certification will review the request and notify the candidate of its determination.

ADMINISTRATIVE PROCEDURES

A. Examination Policies

1. Reexamination Time Frame and Process
   Candidates who fail any part of the examination and wish to retake the failed portion(s) must submit the reexamination form enclosed with the examination scores. Candidates must submit the appropriate fee and their preferred test dates and sites with the form.

2. CPR certification must be current when the retake application is submitted.

3. Candidates must retake failed section(s) of the examination within 1 year of the date of their most recent examination attempt. Failure to retake the examination within this time frame will necessitate the submission of a new application and the candidate will have to retake the entire examination. When submitting a new ap-

plication, the candidate must satisfy all current requirements at the time of application (coursework and clinical hours). The NATABOC recommends that candidates who fail one or more sections of the certification examination review their scores with their endorsing ATC to determine appropriate remedial studies or athletic training experiences, or both.

4. Submission of Required Information

Candidates who are successful on all three sections of the certification examination have **1 year from the date of examination to complete their file of required materials** (e.g., official college transcript). Candidates who do not complete their application within this time frame will have their test results voided and will be required to submit a new application and repeat the certification examination. It is the candidate's responsibility to submit the required application materials.

B. Eligibility Appeal Policy

1. If the NATABOC does not accept an application because of educational or disciplinary reasons, or both, the applicant can appeal the action by writing to the Executive Director of the NATABOC.

2. The appeal must be received at least 60 days before the requested examination date. The applicant is responsible for demonstrating that the appeal should be granted. The Board of Certification will review the request and notify the applicant of its determination.

C. Policies During the Examination Administration

1. A candidate who informs a test site administrator that he or she does not wish to continue taking the portion of the examination currently being administered may not return and complete this portion of the examination later that day. If the candidate retakes the examination at a later date, he or she must submit the retake fee for the portion(s) that were discontinued or not taken.

2. Candidates who arrive late for a portion of the examination may not take that portion of the examination.

3. Disruptive behavior is cause for dismissal from the test site by the test site administrator. No refunds will be given to candidates expelled for disruptive behavior.

4. No visitors (including children) are permitted in testing rooms.

5. Candidates may not bring coats, book bags, luggage, and so forth to their examination desks.

6. Only the individual named on the registration roster will be permitted to take the examination. No substitutions are allowed for registered candidates. Candidates must present valid picture identification at check-in.

7. **Examination misconduct:** Before, during, and after an examination section, all examinees are expected to conduct themselves in an ethical manner and to avoid hampering the ability of fellow examinees around them to perform independently on the examination. Incidents of reported cheating will be investigated by the NATABOC. If a candidate is found to have cheated, that candidate will be barred from taking any NATABOC examination for a period of time to be determined by the NATABOC Professional Practice & Discipline Committee.

D. Failure to Appear

If you fail to appear for one or all sections of the examination, you will forfeit the entire examination fee. Waivers of exam fee forfeiture will be considered in the case of medical emergencies. See Medical or Other Emergencies, which follows, for more information.

E. Medical or Other Emergencies

Waivers of withdrawal penalties or exam fee forfeiture will be considered in the case of medical emergencies. Requests for such waivers must be made in writing and supported by appropriate physician documentation. Requests must be received within 3 weeks after the examination. They will be reviewed on a case-by-case basis.

F. Score Reports

Score reports are mailed via U.S. mail to candidates within 2 to 4 weeks of the examination. No candidate scores will be given by telephone, facsimile transmission, or other electronic means for any reason.

G. Confidentiality

The examination scores are confidential and will not be disclosed unless the NATABOC receives a written request from the candidate or is directed to do so by subpoena or court order. A candidate who wants scores to be released to another entity must indicate in writing which particular scores may be disclosed and identify specifically the person or organization to which the scores should be revealed. No candidate scores will be given by telephone, facsimile transmission, or other electronic means for any reason.

H. Diagnostic Reports

Candidates may receive (for a fee) a diagnostic report of their performance on any section of the certification examination directly from the testing agency. For the written section of the examination, the diagnostic report informs the candidate of the number of correct responses that were selected for the five domains that constitute the written section as well as a breakdown by task statement. The diagnostic report for the simulation informs the candidate of the number of options marked that were Clearly Indicated, Indicated, Neutral, Contraindicated, and Clearly Contraindicated. The report for this test also provides the candidate with information about the number of Contraindicated and Clearly Contraindicated options the candidate appropriately avoided.

A candidate requesting a diagnostic report for the Practical section will receive information about the percentage of the total points possible earned for each problem.

I. Verification of Scores and Appeals

Candidates receiving failing scores may request a rescoring of the answer sheet from the testing agency (for a fee). Information about rescoring will be included with the candidate's score report. On receipt of the request form and fee, the candidate's answer sheet will be hand scored. Requests for rescoring of answer sheets must be received by the testing agency no later than 30 days after the release of the examination results. Requests received later than that will not be processed.

The NATABOC does not encourage candidates whose score is close to passing to request verification of their scores. Because of the procedures used to score and verify scores, it is extremely doubtful that any examination results will change from "fail" to "pass" when rescored.

Improper behavior by a model, examiners, or room proctors and violations of stated examination procedures are acceptable reasons for appealing the results. At the time of the exam, the candidate must inform the test site administrator of any test-related incident that had a negative impact. Next, the candidate must submit written notification of the incident to the NATABOC. This written statement must indicate why the incident negatively affected the candidate's results. The appeal must be received by the NATABOC no later than 30 days after release of examination results. Failure of one or more sections of the certification examination is not an acceptable basis for an appeal.

J. Examination Disclosure

The examination booklets and answer sheets remain the property solely of the NATABOC. These materials are confidential and are not available for review by any person or agency for any reason.

▥ FREQUENTLY ASKED QUESTIONS

Eligibility and Candidate Questions

Where can I find a list of accredited athletic training educational programs?

You will find the list of CAAHEP-accredited programs on the National Athletic Trainers Association (NATA) website (www.nata.org).

I am trying to find a NATABOC-certified athletic trainer to supervise my athletic training experience hours. How can I find someone?

You should contact the local high schools, colleges, and sports medicine clinics. If you still have difficulty, contact the local state athletic training association for assistance. The links to all the state association websites are available on the NATA website at www.nata.org/leadership/district.htm

I just finished a CPR class but have not received my card. I am ready to send in my application. What can I do?

You may submit a letter from the instructor stating that you have completed the course. Your application will be processed. You will not be granted certification until a copy of the card has been received by CASTLE Worldwide, Inc.

Where can I find a copy of the requirements to sit for the exam?

You will find a copy of the requirements in the credentialing information brochure on the NATABOC website. You may also request a copy of the brochure by calling the NATABOC office toll free at 877-BOC-EXAM.

Can I get a waiver for one of the requirements to sit for the exam?

Applicants may submit a written letter of appeal to the NATABOC Board of Directors.

I am applying to sit for the certification examination. How do I determine which of my supervising ATCs should endorse me as a candidate?

The NATABOC-certified athletic trainer who endorses your application must have supervised at least 33 percent of your required 1500 athletic training experience hours.

When submitting my application, do I need to include both my course syllabi and a copy of the course descriptions from my college catalog?

No, either of the two will be accepted.

If I am applying to sit for the certification examination before graduation, are there any special forms that I need to submit with my application?

You must submit written verification of intent to graduate from the dean or department chairperson of the college or university from which you will graduate. If you have not completely satisfied the academic course requirements, you must submit a letter from the college registrar verifying enrollment in the required class(es). Certification will not be issued until an official transcript indicating successful completion of all athletic training coursework and the date of degree is received by CASTLE Worldwide, Inc.

How do I go about getting special accommodations for the exam?

Special circumstances can be accommodated. Please see the Policy for Special Accommodation section, earlier in this chapter.

I have obtained supervised athletic training experience hours in Canada under a CATA-certified athletic therapist. Will these hours count toward the hour requirement for the internship route to certification?

Of the 1500 athletic training experience hours required, 500 may be obtained under the supervision of a CATA-certified athletic therapist.

I received my college degree at an institution in a country other than the United States. Will this fulfill the degree and core course requirements needed to sit for the exam?

You may petition for a substitution of this degree requirement. Such a request will be evaluated at your expense by an independent consultant selected by the NATABOC. The basic and advanced athletic training courses (or the acceptable alternatives) must be successfully completed in a college or university in the United States or be taught by an NATABOC-certified athletic trainer in a foreign college or university for academic credit. The remaining core courses may be accepted from foreign universities as deemed acceptable by the consultant.

How does the 2004 deadline for the elimination of the internship route to certification affect me if I am a current internship athletic training student?

If the application is received by CASTLE Worldwide, Inc., by December 31, 2003, **and** is complete, you will be allowed to sit for the exam in 2004 that is closest to your graduation date. If your application is received and is incomplete or if you have not fulfilled all of the internship section requirements, you will not be permitted to sit for the examination. If you apply to sit for an examination in 2003 but are not given a seat because of exam site capacity, you will be seated for an exam in 2004.

What if I am an internship candidate, and I fail the examination in 2003? Will I be permitted to retake the exam in 2004?

You must retake failed section(s) of the examination within 1 year of the date of your most recent examination attempt. Failure to retake the examination within this time frame necessitates resubmission of a new application, and you must retake the entire examination (all three portions). When submitting a new application, you must satisfy all current requirements at the time of application (coursework and clinical hours). This means that former internship candidates will need to fulfill the curriculum requirements.

After I send in my application to sit for the certification examination, how soon is it processed?

CASTLE Worldwide, Inc., normally processes all applications within 24 hours of receipt.

It is very important for me to have a seat for this next exam. I have been told that all exam sites are at capacity. What can I do?

You may write a letter expressing your concerns with the exam seating policies to the Board of Directors care of the NATABOC office. This does not mean that you will be given a seat.

Is there a waiting list for the examination?

No, there is not a waiting list for the examination.

When are confirmation letters sent?

Confirmation letters are sent out on the day that CASTLE Worldwide, Inc., reserves a seat for you.

How far in advance can I expect to receive my admission ticket for the exam?

Admission tickets are sent out 3 weeks in advance of the exam.

Do you have airline or car rental information for exam candidates?

No. You can obtain better prices on car rentals through individual travel agents. You can find toll-fee numbers for most national car rental agencies in your local yellow pages or online.

May I reschedule my exam?

Yes. You must put your request **in writing** and send it directly to CASTLE Worldwide, Inc. Your request must include your desired test date and site and your signature. There is a $100 rescheduling fee. Fax your request to CASTLE Worldwide, Inc. at (919) 572–6880 or mail it to the address where you sent your application. For more information on rescheduling or to pay the fee by credit card, contact the NATABOC representative at CASTLE Worldwide, Inc. at (919) 572–6880.

When can I expect my score report from my examination?

Score reports are generally sent out 1 to 2 weeks after an examination via the U.S. mail and are sent first class.

Exam Administration Questions

I believe there was an inappropriate occurrence during my exam, how do I file an appeal or grievance?

You must submit a written letter of appeal within **30 days** of your exam. The NATABOC will send you a letter stating that it has received the appeal. Your appeal will be reviewed, and a letter explaining the decision will be sent.

How do I determine if I should call NATA, NATABOC, or CASTLE Worldwide, Inc.

NATABOC answers all credentialing questions. **CASTLE Worldwide, Inc.** answers questions dealing with examination applications. **NATA** answers all questions dealing with membership issues and educational program accreditation.

■ REQUIREMENTS TO MAINTAIN CERTIFICATION

The NATABOC requires that each ATC requalify for certification. At the conclusion of each term, ATCs must meet requirements, including

- Completion of a predetermined number of continuing education units (CEUs), including recertification in CPR at least once in the 3-year term. CPR must be current at the time the CEU report is submitted.
- Adherence to the NATABOC standards of professional practice.
- Submission of annual NATABOC certification fee or payment of NATA annual dues.
- Maintaining the continuing education folder.

Continuing education requirements are meant to ensure that ATCs stay current in the field of athletic training. The purpose of these requirements is to ensure that ATCs continue to

- Obtain current professional development information
- Explore new knowledge in specific content areas
- Master new athletic training-related skills and techniques

- Expand approaches to effective athletic training
- Further develop professional judgment
- Conduct professional practice in an ethical and appropriate manner

The NATABOC has established that all ATCs must obtain a predetermined number of CEUs within a 3-year reporting term. The predetermined amount of CEUs is prorated based on the individual's year of certification. Each individual is also required to submit proof of current CPR certification at least once during the 3-year term. Newly certified athletic trainers will be advised of their continuing education requirements when they receive their certification notice.

The NATABOC has established the following certified status categories: Active, Inactive, Suspended, Voluntarily Resigned, Delinquent, and Revoked.

Certified Status Categories

A. Active Status Policies

1. The minimum number of CEUs required by December 31, 2003, for ATCs who were certified by December 31, 2000, is 80 units; those certified during 2000 will be required to obtain 55 units; and those certified in 2001 will be required to obtain 25 units. Continuing education (recertification) requirements for athletic trainers certified in 2002 will begin with the next continuing education term. The NATABOC will provide all individuals who satisfy their continuing education requirements with a certificate for public display.

2. During the 2000 to 2002 continuing education term, all ATCs, with the exception of those certified in 2002, must obtain at least 5 CEUs by becoming recertified in CPR.

3. Individuals should refer to the 2000 to 2002 NATABOC continuing education file folder for specific guidelines and directions.

4. Failure to satisfy the NATABOC continuing education requirements can result in suspension or revocation of an individual's certification. The status of an ATC who does not satisfy the continuing education requirements by the end of a continuing education term will be changed from active to suspended. If the individual's continuing education requirement has not been met after 6 months from the date of suspension, his or her certification will be revoked.

5. The NATA reimburses the NATABOC for recording and processing continuing education records for its members who were certified by

the NATABOC. ATCs who are not NATA members will be assessed an annual maintenance fee. Nonpayment of this fee can result in a sanction by the NATABOC. The status of an individual who does not pay the annual maintenance fee will be changed to delinquent. An individual whose status is listed as delinquent after February 1 of that year will be changed from delinquent to suspended. If the appropriate fee has not been submitted to the NATABOC by June 1 of the same year, the certification of the ATC will be revoked.

6. An ATC who has had his or her certification revoked must complete the entire entry-level certification process (satisfy current requirements and pass the entry-level certification examination) in order to regain active status.

B. Inactive Policies

1. An ATC who wishes to have his or her certification status changed from active to inactive may make a request through the NATABOC. An application must be submitted to the NATABOC. A $10 nonrefundable application fee must accompany the application each year.

2. Examples of individuals who might desire the inactive status are as follows:
   a. An individual on active military duty or in the Peace Corps
   b. An individual not currently practicing in the field of athletic training
   c. An individual suffering serious medical problems

3. When classified as inactive, the ATC does not have to obtain CEUs.

4. When classified as inactive, the ATC agrees to not do the following:
   a. Serve as a supervisor of students who are satisfying the athletic training requirements for certification eligibility
   b. Serve as a model or examiner for the NATABOC certification examination
   c. Represent himself or herself to the public as a practicing certified athletic trainer or use the initials ATC after his or her name

5. If during a continuing education term an ATC requests to have his or her status changed from inactive to active, he or she will be advised of the number of prorated CEUs required during that term, including proof of current CPR certification.

6. An ATC whose status is classified as inactive for 3 years must attain a passing score on the simulation section of the NATABOC certification examination in order to maintain his or her certified status.

7. An ATC who requests inactive status for 3 years and fails to take and pass the simulation section of the NATABOC certification examination will have his or her status changed to suspended. If the ATC does not pass the simulation section within 1 year of the date of suspension, his or her certification status will be revoked.

8. If an individual wishes to regain his or her certified status following certification revocation, he or she must satisfy the requirements in Section Two: Internship (see p. 7).

C. Suspended

1. An ATC who fails to satisfy the NATABOC continuing education requirements will be suspended. The athletic trainer who is suspended cannot
   a. Serve as a supervisor of students who are satisfying the athletic training requirements for certification eligibility
   b. Serve as a model or examiner for the NATABOC certification examination
   c. Represent himself or herself to the public as a practicing certified athletic trainer or use the initials ATC after his or her name

2. Regulatory agencies, the public, or employers who request to verify the status of an athletic trainer are told only that the suspended athletic trainer is not in good standing.

3. The NATABOC annually sends lists of athletic trainers not in good standing to state regulatory agencies that recognize the NATABOC credential for state licensing and registration purposes.

D. Voluntary Resigned Status Policies

1. An ATC who wishes to voluntarily resign his or her certified status may do so. This status, Resigned, is for those who (1) no longer wish to satisfy the continuing education requirements, (2) no longer wish to pay the NATABOC annual CEU maintenance fee or pay the annual certified membership dues for the NATA, or (3) wish to permanently leave the profession of athletic training.

2. An ATC who voluntarily resigns his or her certification and is therefore classified as Resigned, agrees to not do the following:

a. Serve as a supervisor of students who are satisfying the requirements for certification eligibility

b. Serve as a model or examiner for the NATABOC certification examination

c. Represent himself or herself to the public as a practicing certified athletic trainer or use the initials ATC after his or her name

3. An ATC who voluntarily resigns his or her certified status (NATABOC status Resigned) will be referred to as Retired with the NATA and for other public information purposes.

Addendum: An ATC who has resigned his or her certification may request retired membership status with the NATA membership department. In order to be a retired status candidate a member must have 20 years or more of membership. The request to be changed to retired status must be in writing to the membership department of NATA.

4. An individual classified as resigned who fails to adhere to the previously stated conditions will be subject to the NATABOC standards of professional practice and disciplinary procedures.

For more information on certification examination eligibility, contact CASTLE Worldwide, Inc., the NATABOC, or the NATA. You can visit the NATABOC website at www.nataboc.org, the NATA website at www.nata.org, or the NATA Education Council website at www.cewl.com for more links.

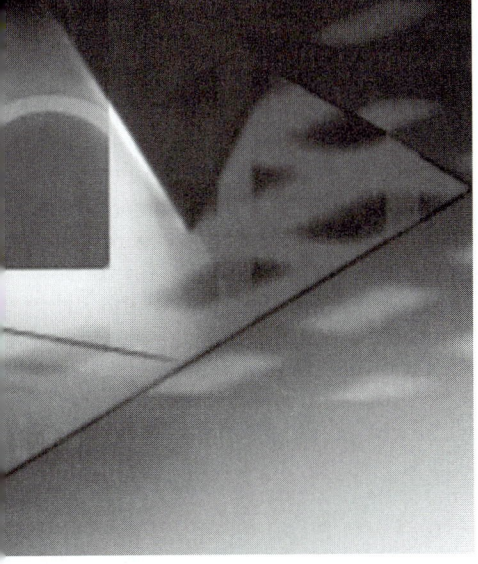

CHAPTER 3

The Certification Examination

The National Athletic Trainers Association Board of Certification (NATABOC) certification examination is administered five times a year at selected sites across the country. As an example, the year 2001 schedule is provided in Table 3–1. For the most recent schedule and sites, contact the NATABOC.

The NATABOC certification examination consists of three separate sections: a written examination, a simulation, and a practical examination. Each of these sections must be successfully completed before certification as an athletic trainer is granted. **Every question in each section of the certification examination is based on the NATABOC, Inc., Role Delineation Study of the Entry-Level Athletic Trainer (Role Delineation).** For more information, see Chapter 4.

▇ RELATED EXAMINATION INFORMATION AND POLICIES

Examination Item Development

Test questions for the certification examination are prepared by committees of certified athletic trainers (ATCs). Each question is validated by three independent judges who are ATCs in item-writing groups; referenced to current resources from the literature on, or related to, athletic training; and repeatedly edited by ATCs for clarity and content. Questions satisfy the test specifications of a Role Delineation Study that was validated by the NATABOC.

Written, simulation, and practical section questions are developed to assess the candidate's knowledge of subject matter from the six domains of athletic training: (1) Prevention; (2) Recognition, Evaluation, and Assessment; (3) Immediate Care (4) Treatment, Rehabilitation, and Reconditioning (5) Organization and Administration; (6) Professional Development and Responsibility. See Table 3–2 for a breakdown of the distribution of written questions by domain as identified by the 1999 Role Delineation Study.

Experts from the NATABOC testing agency also subject each question to editing for grammar and technical adequacy. Thus, content experts who are ATCs write the questions and validate their appropriateness for the examination, and experts in testing review the questions to ensure that the questions perform as intended.

Candidates who have comments about a test question should use the Comment form on their examination booklet cover on the day of the test. The form also allows space for the candidate to explain his or her comments in detail. When item-writing committees meet to revise the examination, they will have information that has been provided by candidates on this form available to them. The Board of Certification, however, will not respond to comments individually.

Passing Point

The passing point used by the NATABOC for the certification examinations is a criterion-referenced approach called the Angoff Modified Technique. Testing professionals consider this technique to be one of the most defensible criterion-referenced methods available for setting passing points. It relies on the pooled judgments of content experts. For example, in this approach, a group of judges who are ATCs are asked to judge each item on the examination. The criterion used to judge each item is, "What is the probability that a minimally acceptable candidate will answer this item correctly?" This question prompts the judges to consider a group of minimally acceptable candi-

TABLE 3–1	NATABOC 2001 CERTIFICATION EXAMINATION SCHEDULE
Examination Date	**Application Deadline**
February 4, 2001	December 29, 2000
April 22, 2001	March 16, 2001
June 10, 2001	May 4, 2001
August 5, 2001	June 29, 2001
November 18, 2001	October 12, 2001

dates and what proportion of that group will answer each item correctly.

The average of the proportions or probabilities is multiplied by the total number of questions on the test. The result then represents the "minimally acceptable" score. The final passing point for the examination is based on this pooled judgment and the calculation of the standard error of the mean. Item analyses for each question and reliability indexes are also calculated for each section of the examination. Each new examination version is equated with the initial or anchor version to ensure that candidates are not rewarded or penalized for taking different versions of the examination.

Examination Scoring

After receiving and checking answer sheets thoroughly for the written and practical sections, the testing service uses sophisticated scanning equipment to create an electronic record of each candidate's responses on the test. A candidate's responses on the simulation section of the examination are manually entered into an electronic storage bank. The testing company uses several security checks to ensure the accuracy of its scoring process, including hand-checking each answer sheet for stray marks or incomplete erasures, scanning answer sheets more than once to compare the results, and randomly choosing answer sheets for hand scoring.

After the examinations are scored, candidates are sent a score report that indicates whether or not they have received a passing score on those sections of the examination they have completed. The score report also indicates the maximum possible scores for those sections, the minimum scores needed to pass, and the actual scores obtained by the candidate.

As of the April 2000 examination administration, 10 unscored items are included in the written examination. Candidates are scored on 140 questions that have been aligned to the test specifications of the Role Delineation Study. Candidate scores will continue to be reported on a scale from 0 to 150 points.

The testing service scores the electronic record for each candidate by comparing the marked responses with the answer key. The total score on the written section of the examination is the number of correct responses. The score on the simulation is calculated according to the scoring key and weights for each option. The practical score is the total number of correct responses adjusted for the weight given each response.

All three sections of the certification examination have proved to be statistically valid and reliable. For more information on the statistical reliability of the NATABOC certification examination, see Appendix C.

◼ THE WRITTEN EXAMINATION

The structure of the written examination is similar to that of other standardized tests. There are 150 multiple-choice questions taken from the six performance domains of athletic training identified by the Role Delineation Study (see Chap. 4). You will have 4 hours to complete this section of the examination (minus whatever time you spend on the practical examination). Each question consists of a **stem** and five possible responses. The stem represents the basic idea, or premise, of the question. Of the five possible responses, **only one is the correct answer;** the other four are incorrect and serve as distractions. These questions are posed in the following formats:

TABLE 3–2	DISTRIBUTION OF WRITTEN QUESTIONS BY DOMAINS IDENTIFIED BY THE 1999 ROLE DELINEATION		
Performance Domain	**Number of Questions**	**Percent of Examination**	
Prevention	23	15%	
Recognition, Evaluation, and Assessment	34	23%	
Immediate Care	32	21%	
Treatment, Rehabilitation, and Reconditioning	33	22%	
Organization and Administration	15	10%	
Professional Development and Responsibility	13	9%	
		1999 Role Delineation Study	

1. Standard A-type questions

   Of the following joints, which one is **proximal** to the knee?

   A. Subtalar
   B. Calcaneocuboid
   C. Tarsometatarsal
   D. Hip
   E. Tibiofibular

   You would select **D** because it is the only articulation above the knee. It is important to note that some questions will test more than one type of knowledge. In this question, two skills are being tested: vocabulary, because the definition of proximal is needed, and anatomy, because knowledge of each of these joints is required.

2. Not-type questions

   Which of the following muscles is **not** located in the lower extremity?

   A. Flexor hallucis longus
   B. Gastrocnemius
   C. Flexor pollicis longus
   D. Peroneus brevis
   E. Plantaris

   In this case, you would have selected **C** because the flexor pollicis longus is a muscle that flexes the thumb.

3. Except-type questions

   All of the following muscles are responsible for movement of the eye **except**

   A. Obliquus inferior bulbi
   B. Levator labii superioris
   C. Rectus inferior bulbi
   D. Rectus medialis bulbi
   E. Rectus superior bulbi

   In this case, you would have selected **B** because the levator labii superioris elevates the upper lip. Note that Except and Not questions are similar in construction: Four of the responses are incorrect, and the other is not.

4. Completion questions

   The biceps brachii is responsible for _____ and _____ of the forearm.

   A. extension and pronation
   B. flexion and pronation
   C. extension and supination
   D. flexion and supination
   E. adduction and circumduction

   In this type of question, your response must complete the sentence to make it true. In this example,

D is the correct response because the two elements in this selection make the stem a correct statement.

5. Multiple correct–type questions

   The muscles of the hamstring group are composed of the

I. Biceps femoris	A. I, II, and III
II. Gracilis	B. II, III, and IV
III. Rectus femoris	C. I, IV, and V
IV. Semimembranosus	D. IV, V, and VI
V. Semitendinosus	E. III, IV, V, and VI
VI. Vastus intermedius	

   In this style of question you would have selected response **C** because the three muscles identified (biceps femoris, semimembranosus, and semitendinosus) compose the hamstring muscle group.

> ### Helpful Hint
>
> The key to answering this type of question correctly is to be certain to identify **all** correct responses from the choices provided and then match them with the list of correct answers.

In the preceding examples there are some questions you may know right away, whereas others require more thought. You may come across a question to which the correct response is immediately apparent, but it is still important that you take your time and fill in the correct response carefully on the answer sheet. When you encounter a more challenging question, context clues can help you arrive at the correct answer.

In some cases, one key phrase or word may separate the correct response from a nearly correct one. Reread the stem and hunt for key terms that may assist you in finding the correct answer. One strategy is to eliminate the obviously incorrect responses to **narrow your choices down** to two or three. Remember, **there is no penalty for guessing in this section of the examination.** If you do not know an answer, guessing is better than leaving it blank. **Do not leave any questions blank.**

During the course of the written examination, you will be faced with three types of questions designed to measure your ability to recall, apply, or analyze information. These three types of questions can be placed on a continuum where **recall** questions are the most basic, **application** questions are the next level, and **analysis** questions represent the most complex type.

Recall questions require only that you remember facts, definitions, rules, and so on. Our first four questions are examples of recall questions.

Application questions require that you apply knowledge to a given situation. For instance, if we were to take question 4 and reword it, it could easily become an application question:

An athlete displays pain and weakness during flexion and supination of the forearm. You would suspect an injury to which muscle?

A. Triceps of the arm
B. Supinator
C. Coracobrachial
D. Anconeus
E. Biceps of the arm

By applying your knowledge of muscle actions to a given set of facts, you would have selected response **E.**

Analysis questions require that you consider more than one piece of information and recognize the relationship between the variables. Expanding on our previous application question, we may further develop it into an analysis question:

An athlete reports to you after a shoulder injury with a marked decrease in right elbow flexion and forearm supination strength and paresthesia along the lateral and medial upper arm, elbow, and forearm. You would suspect impairment of which of the following nerves?

A. Musculocutaneous
B. Axillary
C. Thoracodorsal
D. Median
E. Radial

This question requires that you recognize the muscle involved in the injury, the nerve that innervates it, and the nerve that supplies the dermatome—**A,** the musculocutaneous.

Helpful Hints

To help you with the written portion of the examination, keep the following in mind:

○ There is **only one correct response** per question.

○ **Eliminate inappropriate responses** to narrow down your choices.

○ **Mark each response carefully,** and be certain that the answer number corresponds to the question number.

○ **Do not dwell** on a question if the answer does not come to you immediately. You can return to this question later.

○ There is **no penalty for guessing.**

◢ THE SIMULATION EXAMINATION

The simulation is an interactive examination designed to test your decision-making skills in athletic training. Closely resembling situations you may encounter as an ATC, the simulation requires you to manage various athletic injuries or illnesses, or both. By analyzing a situation and indicating the actions you would take, you progress through questions that test one or more of the six domains of athletic training (see Role Delineation, Chap. 4, or Table 3–2). You have 2½ hours to complete this section of the examination.

This portion of the examination requires the use of two booklets—a problem booklet and an answer booklet—and a latent-image pen. The problem booklet describes the situation and presents the problems to be solved and a list of several possible actions. You mark your responses with the latent-image pen in the answer booklet. Through this mechanism, you know the results of your actions immediately. The answer booklet and latent-image pen are included with this study guide, and a problem booklet containing **sample** problems is found in Chapter 7.

With the exception of numbers, the answer booklet appears to be blank. The ink in the latent-image pen causes the response to become visible. Be careful when choosing your response. **Once you have highlighted your answer, you cannot change it.** Begin highlighting next to the response number and **continue to the right until the double asterisks (**) are reached,** indicating that you have uncovered the entire response (Figure 3–1). (Note: In some responses, you will need to uncover more than one line.)

Helpful Hint

It is not necessary to rub the pen as you would an eraser; rather, rub across the line as if you were highlighting a few words in a textbook. A response that is partially highlighted is taken as a complete response.

The actual simulation consists of eight problems, each containing an opening scene that describes the initial situation facing you and provides various facts regarding the onset of the injury. In some questions, the information presented may represent what you would have seen if you had been covering an event. In other questions, it gives you the basic facts to bring you up to date on the disposition of the injury. Consider the opening scene from the first sample problem in this study guide.

A volleyball player has injured her left ankle during practice. Your evaluation has been completed, and

1.

1. This is

1. This is the highl

1. This is the highlighted response **

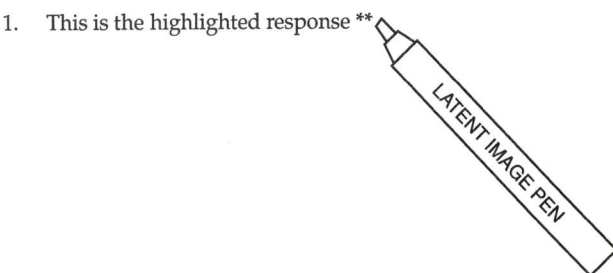

Figure 3–1 Highlighting the latent-image response.

you suspect a moderate second-degree lateral ankle sprain.

Go to Section A

The basic situation has been presented, and you know that (1) the lateral ankle ligaments have been injured, (2) the injury is moderate, and (3) the injury occurred during practice. Based on this information, you are called on to indicate what action(s) you would take. **In the simulation section, unlike the written test, you may need to highlight more than one response for each question.** Now let us examine Section A from the sample question.

Immediately after your evaluation, you will do which of the following? (*Choose only those actions that you have reason to believe are essential to the resolution of the case.*)

1. Tape her ankle securely and see if she can finish practice.
2. Apply ice to the left ankle.
3. Have the athlete walk the injury off.
4. Write a note to excuse her from class tomorrow.
5. Apply a compression wrap to the left ankle.

The sections within a single problem supply various directions and questions about your response to the situation. **The key to success in this portion of the certification examination is to highlight only those responses that are immediately necessary and applicable to provide proper health care for the athlete at that moment.** You are expected to select all options that follow your recommended course of action. Arriving at the final answer via a "shortcut" will detract from the total points you are able to accrue. The ideal

path receives the perfect score. The more you deviate from this path, the more you are penalized. Let us examine the five possible responses from Section A.

1. **Tape her ankle securely and see if she can finish practice.** This response would be contraindicated because the stem indicated that the athlete had a second-degree ankle sprain. You would be risking the athlete's well-being by having her try to practice, which she is unable to do.
2. **Apply ice to the left ankle.** This response is indicated because it is part of the proper protocol in the treatment of an ankle sprain.
3. **Have the athlete walk the injury off.** Reading the highlighted response, it is quite clear that this response is contraindicated: "The athlete cries out in pain when she bears weight." The stem noting that this is a "moderate ankle sprain" should have alerted you to the fact that this was an impractical approach.
4. **Write a note to excuse her from class tomorrow.** Although not an appropriate action, this is a neutral response because it neither helps nor further injures the athlete.
5. **Apply a compression wrap to the left ankle.** This is a clearly indicated response because it is part of the proper ice, compression, and elevation protocol for the treatment of acute injuries.

The proper, or point-earning, responses, were **2** and **5.** If you had chosen response 1 or 3, or both, points would have been deducted from your total. Choosing response 4 would have earned you no points. Note that if you failed to uncover an "indicated" response, your final score would have been reduced. **Also, unlike the case in the written examination, there could be a penalty for guessing if you choose a contraindicated response.**

Helpful Hint
Before marking your responses, read all the possible actions and prioritize the order in which you would do them if you were actually in this situation. Each response is classified as being (from best to worst): (a) indicated, (b) neutral, or (c) contraindicated. Indicated responses earn up to 50 points, whereas contraindicated responses may result in the deduction of up to 50 points. Neutral responses are worth 0 points, so they neither add to nor deduct from your point total. The actual calculation used to score the simulation section uses proficiency and efficiency scores and is very complex and beyond the scope of this study guide.

Uncover the responses in the order that you would actually do them, and pay close attention to

the highlighted responses, because this information further adds to the scenario. Responses may be as simple as "this action is done," indicating that the action you selected has been completed successfully. Other responses, such as to the action "take the athlete's blood pressure," provide significant information regarding the task, for example "100/60 mm Hg and decreasing." If, in this example, you fail to recognize that the athlete is going into shock, it will negatively affect your actions in future sections. In addition, this information can guide you in the current section. For instance, in Section A, the response to "have the athlete walk the injury off" should have alerted you to the fact that returning the athlete to competition was not a safe approach.

Helpful Hint

If you do uncover an inappropriate response, do not panic. The structure of the examination gives some room to recover from errors. **It is STRONGLY ADVISED that you do not go back to previous sections and uncover other responses, because doing so can reduce your point total.**

It is important that you read the current situation and subsequent sections carefully and follow all directions provided. Some sections require only one an-

---

Helpful Hint

The simulation is probably unlike any other examination you have ever taken. You cannot "undo" your actions once they have been selected, and the outcome of the action is immediate. When taking this examination, remember the following:

○ **Carefully read** the opening scene and each problem.

○ **Review all the possible actions** before marking your response(s).

○ **More than one** response may be uncovered.

○ Uncover them **in the order** you would do them in real life.

○ Be careful to **uncover only the desired response(s).**

○ Uncover only those items that are **relevant** to the problem **at that moment.**

○ Remember the selected responses and **use the information** in future responses.

○ There **is a penalty** for guessing if contraindicated responses are chosen.

○ To achieve the maximum point total, **all clearly indicated responses must be uncovered.**

---

swer; others may allow more than one. When you are asked for more than one response, select all responses that you believe are relevant to the circumstances given. You will not receive full credit for the section if you fail to choose a response that is helpful to the case. You will also receive penalties if you select a response that should not have been chosen.

Continue going through the problem section by section until you highlight "End of problem" or another indication that the problem is finished. Some problems will end without a clear outcome or with an outcome other than what you expected. Some problems may end with "The physician supports your decision" or "This is the correct action," but others may end with "The athlete is immediately admitted to the hospital" or "The coach is angry." None of these four finales definitely indicates that you acted either properly or improperly. **If a problem ends with an outcome that surprises or confuses you, do not become overly concerned and certainly do not go back through the problem and attempt to alter the conclusion.**

■ THE PRACTICAL EXAMINATION

The practical examination has been modified and now focuses on the performance of **specific** psychomotor skills. This represents a change from the long-standing format in which a student would essentially conduct a "mock evaluation" of an injury. The practical has also changed in that it no longer **requires** you to explain what you are demonstrating. The practical has evolved in many other ways. Now the examiners can give you some feedback, particularly if you are doing something wrong. There are no longer any trick questions or supplies placed on the table that are not needed. There is always some bias, however, because people are grading your performance. As much as the NATABOC tries to eliminate examiner bias, it still exists and can be a factor in your performance. Learning about the changes in this section and what is now expected can be very beneficial to the candidate.

During the practical examination, candidates are asked to perform a series of specific skills. The examiners then evaluate each response according to the tasks necessary to properly complete the skill. These tasks are based on the psychomotor skills used by entry-level athletic trainers identified by the Role Delineation Study. Examples of the tasks that the candidate may be asked to perform include, but are not limited to, ambulation assists, sensory testing, ligamentous stress tests, special tests, manual muscle tests, taping and wrapping, protective device construction, vital signs, reflex testing, and identification of anatomic landmarks.

Three individuals in addition to the candidate are involved in the testing procedure. One individual serves as the model. He or she will escort you to the examination room and serve as the person on whom you will demonstrate the various tasks. The model may be a man or a woman and will be a certified athletic trainer. However, the model has been trained to act like an athlete. For example, during a question on ankle taping, the model may allow his or her foot to drop into plantar flexion (as an athlete might), which would make it necessary for you to reposition the foot.

Once you are in the examination room, you will find two examiners sitting behind a table. These are the individuals who will actually evaluate your performance. You will be directed to observe a table of supplies. These are at your disposal for use during any portion of the examination. Do not be alarmed if you notice an audiotape recorder in the room. This is provided for your benefit. Your responses are audiotaped, and if there are significant discrepancies between the scores of the two examiners, the NATABOC may elect to review the audiotape.

Helpful Hint

Go ahead and speak. Although you are no longer required to speak during much of this portion of the examination, it may be helpful for you to talk yourself through what you are doing. This can help in three ways. First, it may relax you and keep you on task. Second, it might impress the examiners that you know what you are doing, and why you are doing it. This is something the examiners are trained to avoid, but it can happen anyway. Finally, if one of the examiners missed what you did, the NATABOC can play back the audiotape to hear you describe what you were doing. Obviously, that will not help you if you are not talking.

The practical examination consists of 8 to 14 individual tasks. The room captain will describe each of these tasks one at a time. For instance, the examination may begin with crutch fitting. The room captain would read a task statement such as, *"This task allows you to demonstrate your ability to properly fit an athlete with a pair of crutches. Using the crutches available, please adjust these to fit the model, who has suffered a sprain of the left ankle. You have 4 minutes to complete your response."* At this point, the clock begins, and you should begin your demonstration of crutch fitting. If you are unsure of what is expected of you, ask the room captain to reread the question.

The model is provided for demonstration purposes only. This individual will not answer your questions but will respond to your specific commands (e.g., please hold your arms to your side). As you are completing your task, the examiners will be constantly marking your score sheet. Do not let this distract you because both correct and incorrect scores are indicated on the sheet. In addition, the examiners are instructed to not provide feedback, such as "nicely done" or "good job." This is done to keep the candidates from receiving biased feedback about their performance.

Each section must be completed within the allotted time, and the room captain will stop you when the time is up. Despite the time constraints, **there is adequate time allotted to complete the tasks,** so do not rush through the examination. It is not unusual to complete the scenario in less time than has been provided. If this is the case, tell the examiners "This completes my response."

Helpful Hint

To help you as you move through this examination, keep the following in mind:

○ **Focus** on the assigned task.

○ **Do not rush through the task;** you have plenty of time.

○ **Do not expect feedback** from the model or examiners.

○ The model is there for **demonstration purposes only.**

○ If you are not certain what is expected, **ask the room captain to repeat the question.**

Sources for more information on various topics are included in the following: For questions on policy, discipline, examiner training, and committee work, contact

NATABOC, Inc.
Administrative Office
4223 South 143rd Circle
Omaha, NE 68137
Toll free: 1–877–BOC–EXAM
(262–3926)
Telephone: (402) 559–0091
Fax: (402) 561–0598
E-mail: staff@nataboc.org
Website: www.nataboc.org

For questions on continuing education, change of address, and verification of certification, contact

NATABOC
Continuing Education Office
2952 Stemmons, Suite 200
Dallas, TX 75247
Toll free: 1–800–TRY–NATA (879–6282), ext. 110 or 111
Telephone: (214) 637–2206

For other questions on the profession of athletic training, NATA membership, and educational program accreditation, contact

NATA
2952 Stemmons
Dallas, TX 75247
Toll free: 1–800–TRY–NATA (879–6282)
Telephone: (214) 637–6282
Fax: (214) 637–2206
Fax on demand: (214) 637–6282
Website: www.nata.org

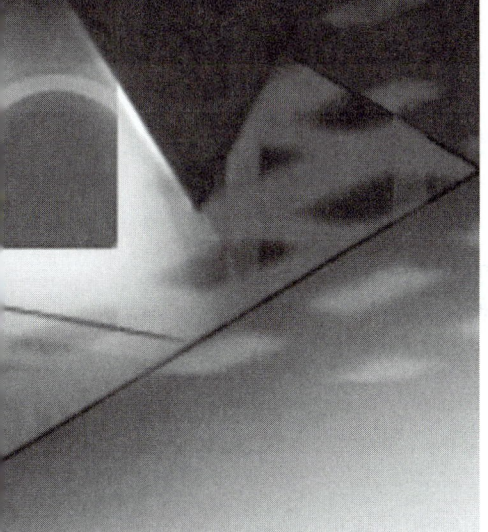

CHAPTER 4

The Role Delineation Study

To be judged valid, a test must relate to some measurable objectives. In college, examinations are given to determine whether a student is proficient in the objectives of a course. Likewise, the National Athletic Trainers Association Board of Certification (NATABOC) examination is administered to determine whether a candidate shows proficiency in the knowledge and skills required to be an athletic trainer. In this model, the Role Delineation Study may be viewed as defining the course objectives.

The Role Delineation Study is an integral part of ensuring that the certification examination is valid. In addition, the Role Delineation Study serves as a job description of a certified athletic trainer (ATC). The study does both of these by ensuring that the questions are valid as to content and that they evaluate the knowledge and abilities needed for someone to function as a competent (entry-level) practitioner. Thus, the NATABOC certification examination protects the public by ensuring that only competent practitioners who have met specific criteria relevant to the practice of athletic training become certified.

This is important because, in addition to being a "blueprint" for the certification examination, the Role Delineation Study describes the areas of knowledge (domains) that are required to work in the profession.

This "scope of practice" identifies knowledge, skills, and abilities required for athletic training in every setting and at every level. It is interesting to note how the domains of the Role Delineation Study have changed over the years. Observing the changes in the study over time (Tables 4–1 through 4–4) provides us with a historical perspective of how our profession has changed (in addition to what has changed on the certification examination).

The changes in the number of domains and also how the 1995 Role Delineation study identified "universal competencies," or overlapping areas of knowledge, are shown in Table 4–2. To explain the concept of universal competencies, consider "Athletic Training Evaluation." Knowledge of evaluation skills is not limited to the assessment of an acute injury. Athletic trainers are also required to identify the presence of predisposing conditions (Prevention) and follow-up evaluations used to assess the stage of healing and the efficacy of the treatment and rehabilitation program (Rehabilitation and Reconditioning). Furthermore, the athletic trainer must be able to document these findings sufficiently (Health Care Administration) and fulfill an obligation to remain up-to-date with current evaluation skills, knowledge, and techniques (Professional Development and Responsibility).

TABLE 4–1	1999 NATABOC ROLE DELINEATION STUDY, 4TH EDITION
Domain I: Prevention	
Domain II: Recognition, Evaluation, and Assessment	
Domain III: Immediate Care	
Domain IV: Treatment, Rehabilitation, and Reconditioning	
Domain V: Organization and Administration	
Domain VI: Professional Development and Responsibility	

TABLE 4–3	1990 NATABOC ROLE DELINEATION STUDY, 2ND EDITION
Domain 1: Prevention (preparticipation, environment, equipment)	
Domain 2: Recognition and Evaluation	
Domain 3: Management/Treatment and Disposition	
Domain 4: Rehabilitation	
Domain 5: Organization and Administration	
Domain 6: Education and Counseling	

TABLE 4–2	1995 NATABOC ROLE DELINEATION STUDY, 3RD EDITION
Performance Domains	
Domain 1: Prevention of Athletic Injuries	
Domain 2: Recognition, Evaluation, and Immediate Care of Athletic Injuries	
Domain 3: Rehabilitation and Reconditioning of Athletic Injuries	
Domain 4: Health Care Administration	
Domain 5: Professional Development and Responsibility	
Universal Competencies (That Transcend Domains)	
1. Domain-Specific Content	
2. Athletic Training Evaluation	
3. Human Anatomy	
4. Human Physiology	
5. Exercise Physiology	
6. Biomechanics	
7. Psychology/Counseling	
8. Nutrition	
9. Pharmacology	
10. Physics	
11. Organization and Administration	

TABLE 4–4	1982 NATABOC ROLE DELINEATION STUDY OF THE ENTRY-LEVEL ATHLETIC TRAINER
Domain 1: Prevention (preparticipation, environment, equipment)	
Domain 2: Recognition and Evaluation	
Domain 3: Management/Treatment and Disposition	
Domain 4: Rehabilitation	
Domain 5: Organization and Administration	
Domain 6: Education and Counseling	

For more information on the latest role delineation study, contact the NATABOC.

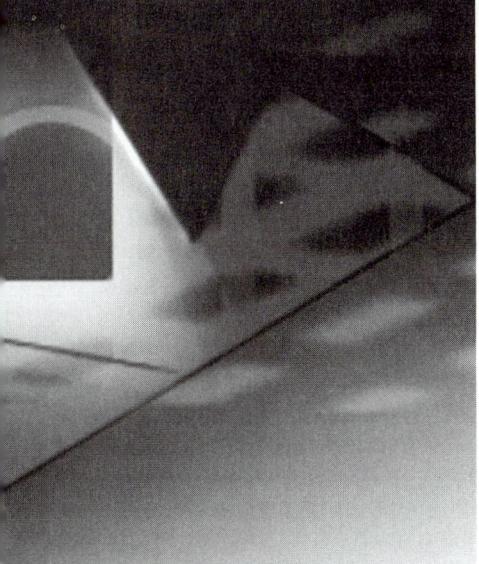

CHAPTER 5

Preparing for the Examination

You began preparing for this examination the first time you set foot in an athletic training class or an athletic training room or covered a practice or game. The certification examination reflects the culmination of your knowledge and clinical skills, but this is not to say that you cannot prepare for it. Because the examination is made up of many sections, and because the Role Delineation Study covers such a broad scope, no one source should be relied on to adequately cover all topics. The reference list used in constructing the certification examination is included in Appendix D of this study guide. Because the Role Delineation Study plays an integral role in the development of the test, it is an excellent guide for preparing for the content areas of the examination.

You should review the Role Delineation Study and, as you read each competency, rate yourself on a scale of 1 to 10. Be honest with yourself, and think back to how much formal education you received on each topic. You may also want to consider the quality of the instruction. We have all had bad teachers or instructors who have skipped a chapter in a book or a section of a course. You may also have been absent (or otherwise preoccupied) on the day when a certain topic was covered. After you have rated your perceived knowledge on each competency (knowledge) and skill, go back and review your rankings. If you do a good job and read each specific competency, know what it means, and rate yourself on it, this could be a great blueprint of what you need to study. You know better than anyone else what information you have mastered and what you have not. We all forget information and need a refresher course. If you are honest with yourself, you will be able to identify your weaknesses and correct them before challenging the certification examination.

In this chapter we will discuss how to prepare for each section of the certification examination and will provide various strategies. The right frame of mind is essential for success on the test. Rather than studying for the National Athletic Trainers Association Board of Certification (NATABOC) certification examination, this process may be viewed as "refreshing" your knowledge. Likewise, the examination itself should not be viewed as an obstacle but rather as an opportunity to demonstrate your knowledge of athletic training. You should have been exposed to a significant amount of the information that will appear on the examination during the course of your classroom education and practical experience. The certification examination will measure your knowledge from a wide range of content areas just like a "comprehensive examination." Preparing for this examination refreshes the knowledge you have already gained. This study guide can help you to do this and to identify areas of weakness, but it is not designed to teach you all of the domains and content of athletic training.

It is best to begin this process well in advance of the test date. "Cramming" information just before the examination is discouraged because it could result more in confusion than in learning. You should start early, but do not take the test before you are ready. Students are often anxious to take the examination as soon as they are eligible, but being eligible is not the same as being prepared. Taking the examination before you are prepared could result in failure in one or more sections and does nothing to help your confidence, your motivation to study more, or your bank balance. Wait until you have had sufficient time to prepare for the examination, even if that means delaying the examination date or choosing a less convenient site.

Carefully going through the sample problems in this guide is an excellent way to start the refreshing process. Evaluate the questions that gave you trouble and focus a significant portion of your attention in these areas. Many students tend to study and reread the topics that most interest them and that they already understand and avoid the less understood topics. Obviously, this does not help the learning process and should be avoided. Try to stay focused on improving the areas in which you are weak.

You should study one good modalities book (such as Starkey's *Therapeutic Modalities*), one good evaluation book (such as Starkey and Ryan's *Evaluation of Orthopedic and Athletic Injuries,* 2nd edition), and one good all-around book (such as Arnheim and Prentice's *Principles of Athletic Training*). Do not study two modalities books. Every book disagrees in some aspects with other books, and this will only confuse you.

This study guide provides you with sample questions to orient you to the three sections that you will encounter when you sit for the NATABOC examination. It is recommended that you take these sample examinations under conditions that closely resemble actual test conditions. That is, you should time yourself, not use any extra material, and resist the temptation to look up an answer to a question until you have completed the practice test.

▮ PREPARING FOR THE WRITTEN EXAMINATION

There are many resources available to begin refreshing your knowledge for this portion of the examination. You may wish to take the written examination provided in this study guide first and then score it to determine your strengths and weaknesses. If you guess at a question or labor to arrive at a conclusion, make note of this on your answer sheet and consider it a weakness. Although you should not disregard your areas of strength totally, most of your studying should focus on your weaker areas. There is little point to rereading information that you have already mastered.

Your study habits should not focus only on the exact questions you missed. Rather, you should focus your attention on the content area of the question. Simply finding the correct answer to a single question will do little to strengthen your knowledge in the entire subject area. Keep in mind that this is only a sample examination and that you will not see the same questions on the actual examination.

Perhaps the best place to begin refreshing your memory is with old class notes. These can provide a concise overview of the necessary information, and your ability to recall this knowledge can be enhanced by seeing the information in your own handwriting. If you still have old tests from therapeutic modalities, injury prevention, exercise physiology, nutrition, and other athletic training content areas, try retaking the tests or find the correct answers to questions that you missed. Many athletic training educators have old tests on file for this purpose, so these would be good resources for your review.

Of course, textbooks are an invaluable resource in preparing for the written examination. However, the questions that make up the written examination are on a wide range of topics and are derived from many sources (see Appendix D). With this in mind, it is highly unlikely that one textbook will adequately provide the scope and depth required to successfully challenge the examination. If you find, for example, that rehabilitation questions were not your strong point, you may wish to use a textbook dedicated solely to that topic or focus on the rehabilitation section in one of the more broadly scoped books (such as that by Arnheim and Prentice). However, you should not use more than one book on a topic; different books say things differently, which can cause even more confusion.

Helpful Hints

Your preparation for the written section of the examination will prepare you for the other sections as well. The material is all athletic training! Everyone says that one section of the examination is more difficult than the others, but not everyone agrees on which section is hardest. I believe that this is a right brain versus left brain issue. Some people are more visual and artistic; others are more analytical. The same is true for the certification examination. Some people prefer the written section, others prefer the practical, and still others prefer the simulation section. However, it is all athletic training knowledge, so it is just a matter of how you prefer to receive the questions. Do not become stressed about a particular section. Instead, remind yourself that it is just athletic training knowledge, which you already possess.

▮ PREPARING FOR THE SIMULATION EXAMINATION

The simulation section is perhaps the most difficult portion of the examination to prepare for because it relies heavily on decision-making skills. The sample problems provided in this study guide will familiarize you with the mechanical and thought processes involved in taking this portion of the examination. In addition, there are computer software packages available that operate similarly to the simulation section. These could also be very beneficial in acquainting you with this type of examination.

If you make errors in the sample problems provided in this study guide, try to understand why the errors occurred. Some individuals require large amounts of information before making a decision, which does not always correspond well with the simulation. If this is the case with you, remember to choose only those responses that are immediately necessary to provide proper care for the athlete. Conversely, other individuals are too hasty in their decisions or try to reveal as few responses as possible. Try to determine where you fit in this continuum by using the sample questions in this study guide. If you have a tendency to reveal too many responses on the practice test in this study guide, chances are you may do the same during the actual certification examination.

Your preparation for the other sections of this examination should also help you prepare for the simulation section. The cognitive knowledge gained in studying for the written section will aid you in determining what actions are appropriate and why. Preparing for the practical examination may also assist you in reinforcing your decision-making process and in the sequencing of events.

PREPARING FOR THE PRACTICAL EXAMINATION

The practical examination tests your psychomotor skills, those parts of athletic training that require you to use manual techniques. With this in mind, the practical section of the certification examination will call on your hands-on skills. These psychomotor skills are identified in the Role Delineation Study.

Preparation for this portion of the examination involves both knowledge of the skills being tested and comfort in performing these skills in front of critical judges. Arrange to practice these skills with your peers and in front of certified athletic trainers (ATCs); you should be given a series of tasks and a set amount of time in which to complete your response.

Helpful Hints

Performing these in front of an "audience" helps to acclimate you to being judged on your actions, and you will receive valuable feedback regarding possible areas of improvement. The realism of these practice sessions can be increased if people you do not know evaluate you.

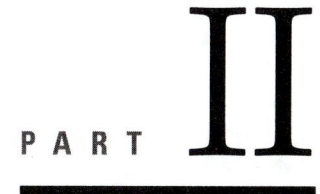

Sample
Examinations

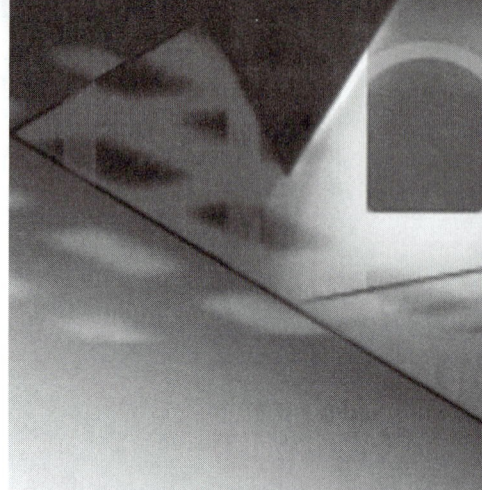

CHAPTER 6

The Written Examination

WRITTEN EXAMINATION INFORMATION

Figures 6–1 and 6–2 are examples of the type of answer sheets used for certification examinations. It is important to mark your answer on the correct line and in the correct column. You are advised to answer every question because your final score will be determined by the number of questions you answer correctly. There is no penalty for guessing on this section of the examination. Remember to use only a number 2 pencil to shade in the correct answer and to erase all stray marks completely.

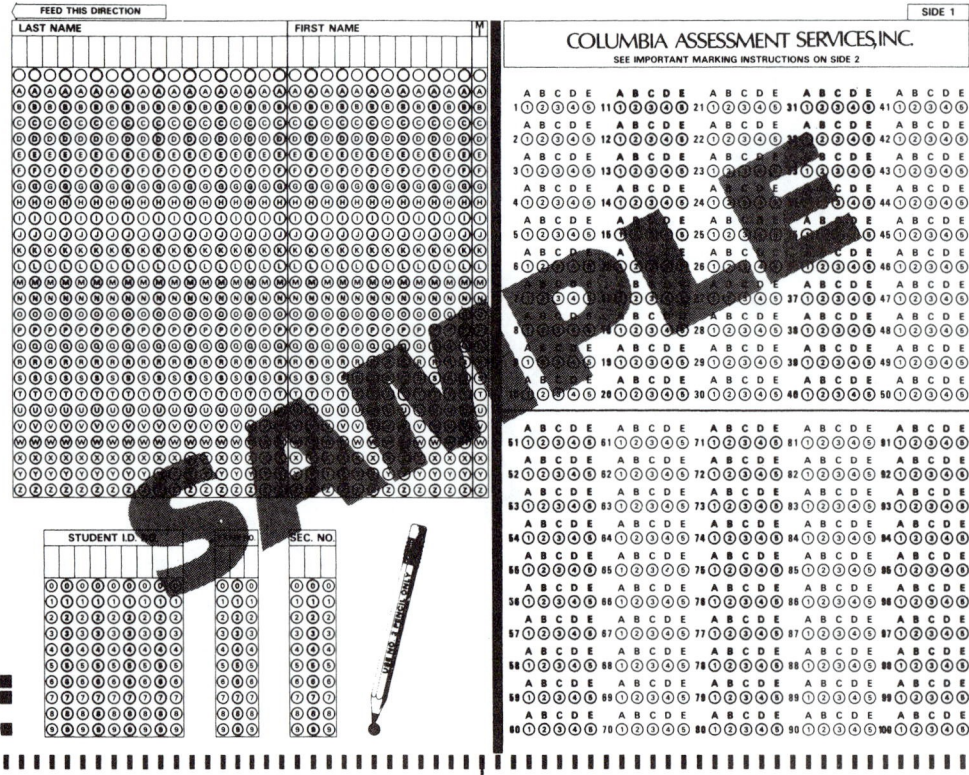

Figure 6–1 Scantron Sheet, 2nd ed., p. 76 (From CASTLE Worldwide, Inc., formerly Columbia Assessment Services [CAS], Inc.).

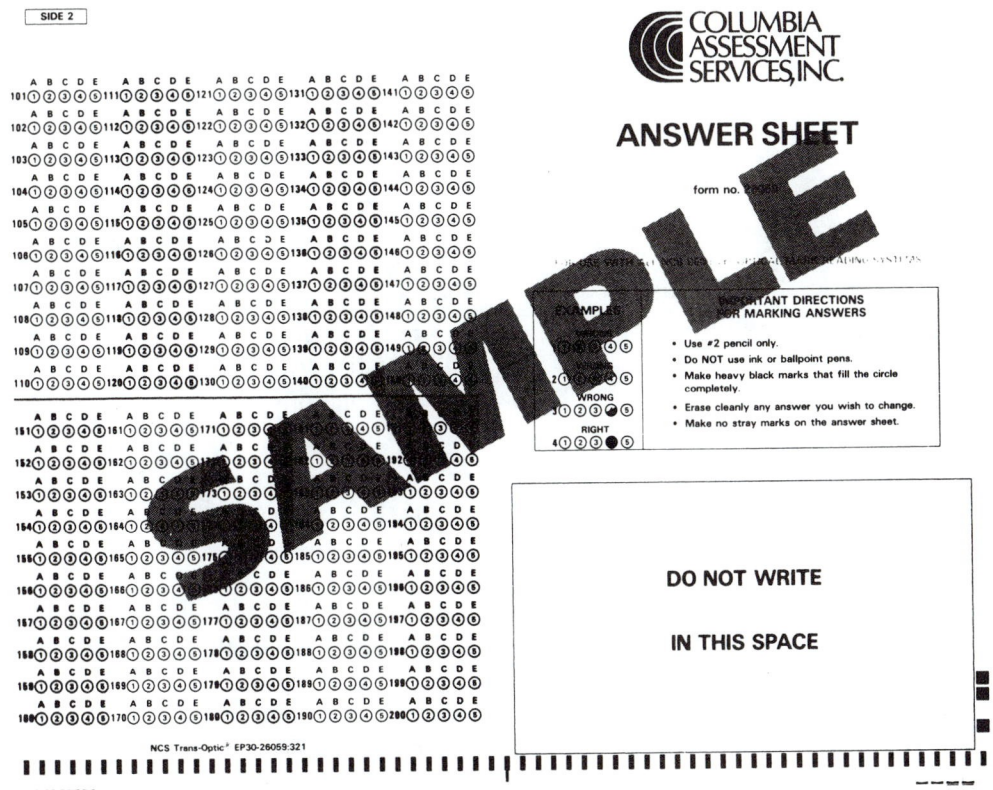

Figure 6–2 Scantron Sheet, 2nd ed., p. 77 (From CASTLE Worldwide, Inc., formerly Columbia Assessment Services [CAS], Inc.).

SAMPLE WRITTEN QUESTIONS

DOMAIN I: PREVENTION

1. The best health care begins with
   A. Prevention.
   B. Careful diagnosis.
   C. Adequate drug therapy.
   D. Modern medical instruments.
   E. More surgical techniques.

2. The bat swing in baseball (movement of the arms) takes place in which of the following planes?
   A. Frontal
   B. Transverse
   C. Sagittal
   D. Reverse
   E. Supine

3. During the menstrual cycle, the disintegration of the endometrial lining as a result of fallen levels of estrogen and progesterone begins on which day of the menstrual cycle?
   A. 1st day
   B. 4th day
   C. 18th day
   D. 25th day
   E. 35th day

4. The forearm extensor muscles during a push-up are
   A. Prime movers.
   B. Antagonists.
   C. Synergists.
   D. Stabilizers.
   E. Contractors.

5. The least reliable source of vitamin C among the following is a/an
   A. Raw tomato.
   B. Orange juice.
   C. Grapefruit half.
   D. Cooked cabbage.
   E. Fresh strawberries.

6. The contraction of the abdominal muscles during the push-up is an example of
   A. Isometric contraction.
   B. Isotonic contraction.
   C. Concentric contraction.
   D. Eccentric contraction.
   E. Continuous contraction.

7. The term *medial* refers to which of the following?
   A. Toward the head
   B. Toward the midline of the body
   C. Toward the trunk
   D. Back portion of the body
   E. Away from the trunk

8. The vertebral border of the spine of the scapula aligns with the spinous process of which vertebra?
   A. C8
   B. T1
   C. T2
   D. T3
   E. T4

9. The jump shot in basketball (movement of the criterion arm) is done in which plane?
   A. Frontal
   B. Sagittal
   C. Transverse
   D. Medial
   E. Lateral

10. Arm action during the elementary backstroke is done in which plane?
    A. Frontal
    B. Sagittal
    C. Transverse
    D. Reverse
    E. Supine

11. The diencephalon is formed by the following structures: _____.
    A. Meninges and meningeal arteries
    B. Choroid plexuses and venous sinuses
    C. Falx of cerebrum and the falx of cerebellum
    D. Pons, medulla oblongata, and circle of Willis
    E. Thalamus, hypothalamus, and epithalamus

12. Movement for a right-handed individual to tighten a screw with a screwdriver relates to which motion?
    A. Rotation
    B. Pronation
    C. Supination
    D. Circumduction
    E. Adduction

13. A muscle that adds limited force for a given movement is a/an
    A. Prime mover.
    B. Antagonist.
    C. Synergist.
    D. Stabilizer.
    E. Resister.

14. The ulna in extension of the arm is an example of a
    A. First-class lever.
    B. Second-class lever.
    C. Third-class lever.
    D. Fourth-class lever.
    E. Fifth-class lever.

15. Which bone is not found in the hand or wrist?
    A. Navicular
    B. Talar
    C. Lunate
    D. Triquetral
    E. Trapezium

16. The motion of the legs during running is
    A. Rotary.
    B. Curvilinear.
    C. Rectilinear.
    D. Perpendicular.
    E. Continuous.

17. Sodium cation (Na$^+$) movement to the inside of a neuron following a stimulus is responsible for the
    A. −70 mV resting membrane potential.
    B. +30 mV peak of the action potential.
    C. Repolarization of the membrane.
    D. Hyperpolarization of the membrane.
    E. Hypopolarization of the membrane.

18. The motion of the head through space while running in a straight line should be
    A. Rotary.
    B. Curvilinear.
    C. Rectilinear.
    D. Perpendicular.
    E. Continuous.

19. The force that a bat expends on the hands while swinging at a ball is
    A. Moment of force.
    B. Centripetal force.
    C. Centrifugal force.
    D. Summation of force.
    E. Distal force.

20. The iliopsoas (iliac and psoas major) primarily acts in hip
    A. Flexion.
    B. Extension.
    C. Abduction.
    D. Adduction.
    E. Supination.

21. The sequential application of the velocities of the hips, shoulders, and arms while executing the tennis forehand drive is an example of
    A. Summation of forces.
    B. Trading distances for forces.
    C. Angular and linear velocity change with length of lever.
    D. Greatest linear velocity perpendicular to axis of rotation.
    E. Moment of force.

22. Unequal pupil size is also referred to as
    A. Anisocoria.
    B. Astigmatism.
    C. Myopia.
    D. Nystagmus.
    E. Hypertrophia.

23. When lifting a 40-pound suitcase from the street into an automobile trunk, you should have bent knees, a straight back, and bent elbows because
    A. That will afford opportunity for greater muscle contraction in the upper arm.
    B. The back muscles are stronger.
    C. This position offers less resistance to the waist.
    D. This position supports the muscles used to lift heavier objects.
    E. The knees can support more weight than the elbow can.

24. Which of the following has the opposite action of a prime mover?
    A. Stabilizer
    B. Choice mover
    C. Supporting muscles
    D. Neutralizer
    E. Antagonists

25. Which of the following eliminates unwanted action?
    A. Stabilizer
    B. Mover
    C. Supporting muscles
    D. Neutralizer
    E. Antagonists

26. Which of the following holds the body erect against the pull of gravity?
    A. Stabilizer
    B. Mover
    C. Supporting muscles
    D. Neutralizer
    E. Antagonists

27. Osmosis functions by having
    A. A semipermeable membrane that is permeable to more than one substance.
    B. A membrane that is semipermeable to only one substance.
    C. A membrane that is semipermeable to water and other substances.
    D. A membrane that is semipermeable to water.
    E. A membrane that is permeable to water and other substances.

28. Epithelial tissue has a function of
    A. Protection, absorption, and secretion.
    B. Support, protection, and transportation.
    C. Communication, protection, and support.
    D. Elimination, support, and communication.
    E. Protection, support, and elimination.

29. The magnitude of muscular force available in a muscle is in direct proportion to
    A. Number and size of fibers.
    B. Pain threshold.
    C. Length of fibers.
    D. Elasticity of fibers.
    E. Number of antagonists.

30. Which muscle is not part of the rotator cuff?
    A. Supraspinous
    B. Infraspinous
    C. Teres minor
    D. Teres major
    E. Subscapular

31. The smaller pectoral, latissimus dorsi, and infraspinous muscles perform what shoulder motion?
    A. Flexion
    B. Extension
    C. Abduction, glenohumeral
    D. Adduction, glenohumeral
    E. Stabilization

32. The sensation of warmth relates to a/an
    A. Chemoreceptor.
    B. Electromagnetic receptor.
    C. Thermoreceptor.
    D. Mechanoreceptor.
    E. Sensitoreceptor.

33. The rhomboid and anterior serratus muscles perform which scapular motion?
    A. Elevation
    B. Depression
    C. Downward rotation
    D. Upward rotation
    E. Stabilization

34. The T wave of the normal electrocardiogram (ECG) occurs before the
    A. Closing of the atrioventricular (AV) valves.
    B. Opening of the aortic valves.
    C. Closing of the aortic valves.
    D. First heart sound.
    E. Opening of the AV valves.

35. The teres minor muscle performs what motion at the shoulder?
    A. Adduction, scapular
    B. Abduction, scapular
    C. Internal rotation
    D. External rotation
    E. Stabilization

36. The middle deltoid muscle performs what motion?
    A. Flexion
    B. Extension
    C. Abduction, glenohumeral
    D. Adduction, glenohumeral
    E. Stabilization

37. Diffusion operates by having
    A. A semipermeable membrane that is permeable to more than one substance.
    B. A membrane that is semipermeable to only one substance.
    C. A membrane that is semipermeable to water and other substances.
    D. A membrane that is permeable to water.
    E. A membrane that is semipermeable to water.

38. The gallbladder has the function of
    A. Digestion with enzymes.
    B. Storage of bile.
    C. Secretion of insulin.
    D. Hormone production for carbohydrate metabolism.
    E. Secretion of glucose.

39. The contraction of the forearm extensors while the body is going up and down, as when doing a pull-up, is an example of
    A. Isometric contraction.
    B. Isotonic contraction.
    C. Concentric contraction.
    D. Eccentric contraction.
    E. Motor contraction.

40. The muscles of the anterior chest wall that aid in the movement of a push-up are
    A. Prime movers.
    B. Antagonists.
    C. Synergists.
    D. Stabilizers.
    E. Neutralizers.

41. The major problem to overcome in fat digestion is the
    A. Acquisition of sufficient surface area for aqueous enzymes to perform fat digestion.
    B. Extreme solubility of fats in watery solutions.
    C. Emulsification of large quantities of highly saturated fatty acids.
    D. Breakdown of large fat droplets to chylomicrons.
    E. Viscous nature of fat in the aqueous environment of the stomach.

42. The sensation of taste relates to a/an
    A. Chemoreceptor.
    B. Electromagnetic receptor.
    C. Thermoreceptor.
    D. Mechanoreceptor.
    E. Sensitoreceptor.

43. To catch a swiftly thrown softball with the least danger of injury, one should
    A. Receive the impact of the ball with the hands.
    B. "Give" with the hands and step backward in order to reduce the force of the impact.
    C. Step backward and keep the arms extended so the shock of the impact is absorbed.
    D. Step forward and keep the arms extended so the shock of the impact is absorbed.
    E. Lean into the ball to absorb the force of the impact with the entire body.

44. The horizontal position is employed in all swimming strokes because
    A. It is easier to use both arms and legs in that position.
    B. The body encounters less water resistance in the horizontal position.
    C. It permits more water to be displaced.
    D. It promotes buoyancy.
    E. It prevents stress on the joints in the horizontal position.

45. When one is attempting to hit a pitched softball as far as possible, which of the following pitches should one choose to hit?
    A. A slow ball, because there is less velocity to overcome, thus permitting more speed and distance
    B. A fast ball, because the bat must have less acceleration than the ball on impact to achieve the desired distance
    C. A fast ball, because the greater velocity of the ball combined with the velocity of the bat will produce the best chance for achieving the desired distance
    D. A slow ball, because there is more time to prepare the body for the force it will need to overcome
    E. A fast ball, because the bat must encounter more acceleration than the ball on impact to achieve the desired distance

46. Dorsal interosseous muscles cause extension and _____ of metacarpophalangeal (MCP) joints.
    A. Flexion
    B. Extension
    C. Abduction
    D. Adduction
    E. Supination

47. Volar interosseous muscles cause flexion and _____ of MCP joints.
    A. Flexion
    B. Extension
    C. Abduction
    D. Adduction
    E. Supination

48. The lumbrical muscles cause flexion of the MCP joints and _____ of interphalangeal (IP) joints.
    A. Flexion
    B. Extension
    C. Abduction
    D. Adduction
    E. Supination

49. The radial extensor muscles of the wrist and the radial flexor muscles of the wrist working together cause which motion of the wrist and forearm?
    A. Flexion
    B. Extension
    C. Abduction
    D. Adduction
    E. Supination

50. The biceps muscle of the arm causes _____ at the radioulnar joint.
    A. Flexion
    B. Extension
    C. Abduction
    D. Adduction
    E. Supination

51. The greatest gluteus muscle primarily acts in hip
    A. Flexion.
    B. Extension.
    C. Abduction.
    D. Adduction.
    E. Supination.

52. The quadriceps muscle of the thigh, as a group, primarily acts in knee
    A. Flexion.
    B. Extension.
    C. Abduction.
    D. Adduction.
    E. Supination.

53. The gastroesophageal sphincter
    A. Serves to regulate the movement of swallowed materials into the stomach.
    B. Serves to prevent stomach contents from being forced back into the esophagus.
    C. Is represented by the first 4 cm of the esophagus.
    D. Is also called the pyloric sphincter.
    E. Is found at the junction between the stomach and the small bowel.

54. Calculate the energy value of this meal:

FOOD	PROTEIN	FAT	CHO
One hamburger	17 g	22 g	40 g
One large cola			25 g
One order French fries	4 g	14 g	40 g

    The total calories in the meal were
    A. 162.
    B. 189.
    C. 345.
    D. 828.
    E. 945.

55. Which nutrient requires gastric intrinsic factor for absorption?
    A. Calcium
    B. Vitamin B_{12}
    C. Vitamin A
    D. Iron
    E. Vitamin D

56. In general terms, metabolism consists of basically two types of biochemical reactions. These include
    A. Activation reactions and energy-trapping reactions.
    B. Isomerase reactions and mutase reactions.
    C. Degradative reactions and synthetic reactions.
    D. Oxidation reactions and reduction reactions.
    E. Productive reactions and reduction reactions.

57. Deficiencies of this vitamin usually occur only in newborn infants, persons taking certain drugs, or people with faulty fat absorption.
    A. Vitamin D
    B. Vitamin K
    C. Vitamin B_{12}
    D. Folic acid
    E. Vitamin A

58. The hamstrings cause knee
    A. Flexion.
    B. Extension.
    C. Abduction.
    D. Adduction.
    E. Supination.

59. Production of carbon involves
    A. Glycolysis.
    B. Krebs cycle.
    C. Electron transport chain.
    D. Glycogen formation.
    E. Enzymatic release.

60. Electrons that are exchanged among organic compounds during oxidation/reduction reactions undergo their largest energy changes in
    A. Glycolysis.
    B. The electron transport chain.
    C. The Krebs cycle.
    D. The Cori cycle.
    E. The Starling cycle.

61. Anemia is not caused by
    A. Lack of intrinsic factor.
    B. Lowered oxygen carrying capacity.
    C. Cobalt deficiency.
    D. Lack of folic acid.
    E. Iodine deficiency.

62. To prevent the transmission of bloodborne pathogens such as hepatitis B virus or human immunodeficiency virus, universal precautions must be taken with which of the following?
    A. Sweat
    B. Urine
    C. Feces
    D. Tears
    E. Any unidentified fluid

63. Oxidation is a sequence of reactions releasing two carbon units from fatty acids in the form of
    A. Depressed fat metabolism, which cannot supply energy when glucose is scarce.
    B. Accumulated insulin in the bloodstream without carbohydrate for it to act on.
    C. Acetylcoenzyme A.
    D. Oxaloacetic acid.
    E. Pyruvic acid.

64. The bladder has a function of
    A. Establishing acid-base relationships.
    B. Being a reservoir for urine.
    C. Being a reservoir for urine and helping to expel urine.
    D. Collecting urine and establishing acid-base relationships.
    E. Accumulating electrolytes before urination.

65. The medical term for "tennis elbow" is
    A. Lateral humeral epicondylitis.
    B. Medial humeral epicondylitis.
    C. Radial tunnel syndrome.
    D. Ulnar tunnel syndrome.
    E. Ulnar epicondylitis.

66. The term *inferior* refers to which of the following?
    A. Toward the feet
    B. Away from the midline of the body
    C. Away from the trunk
    D. Front portion of the body
    E. Toward the midline of the body

67. Action potentials of nerves do not undergo summation when muscles contract. Summation of action potentials is prevented by
    A. Low membrane permeability of sodium.
    B. The absolute refractory period.
    C. The action of the sodium pump.
    D. Rapid depletion of acetylcholine.
    E. Increased membrane permeability of sodium.

68. An electroencephalograph is a
    A. Recording of electrical activity of the heart.
    B. Recording of electrical activity in the brain.
    C. Machine used to reward monkeys for making correct choices.
    D. Machine used to measure muscle tension during isometric contraction.
    E. Machine used to record the muscular activity of the heart.

69. For conditioning a baseball pitcher, the phase in which the emphasis should be on significant gains in strength is which of the following?
    A. Off season is the best.
    B. In season is the best.
    C. Preseason is the best.
    D. Year-round emphasis is the best.
    E. Rapid strength gains are to be avoided in pitchers.

70. Which of the following is not an essential component of the simple reflex arc?
    A. Sensory neuron
    B. Receptor
    C. Effector muscle or gland
    D. Brain
    E. Motor neuron

71. Diabetic coma results from
    A. Oversecretion of insulin.
    B. Lack of sufficient insulin.
    C. Low blood glucose level.
    D. Tubular load exceeding the maximal tubular excretory capacity of the kidneys (T_m).
    E. Digestion of too much sugar.

72. Two enzymes capable of completing protein digestion in the small intestine are
    A. Pancreatic amylase and salivary amylase.
    B. Pancreatic lipase and bile salts.
    C. Pepsin and trypsin.
    D. Carboxypeptidase and aminopeptidase.
    E. Bile salts and salivary amylase.

73. Creatine phosphate in muscles can best be described as
    A. A high-energy storage compound used to regenerate adenosine triphosphate (ATP).
    B. A high-energy compound that can substitute for ATP once ATP is depleted.
    C. A high-energy storage compound that is not depleted even during vigorous exercise.
    D. A waste product that builds up in muscle during strenuous exercise.
    E. A source of energy constantly burned along with ATP to generate more intensity during exercise.

74. During extreme oxygen debt
    A. All sources of ATP are depleted and fatigue is usually apparent.
    B. ATP is still available through reaction with creatine phosphate.
    C. ATP can still be produced through metabolic pathways that do not require oxygen.
    D. ATP is converted into glycogen and can be stored in the liver.
    E. Additional ATP is activated by calcium ions (Ca^{++}).

75. The term *anticoagulation* is most closely associated with
    A. Lymphoid tissue.
    B. Bradycardia.
    C. Erythrocytes.
    D. Heparin.
    E. Lymphocytes.

76. Bradycardia refers to
    A. Increased heart rate.
    B. Decreased heart rate.
    C. Erratic heart rate.
    D. Increased stroke volume.
    E. Decreased cardiac output.

77. Target organ specificity refers to
    A. The ability of hormones to travel to localized areas in the body.
    B. The fact that usually only specific areas in the body are sensitive to a given hormone and thus its effect is seen there.
    C. The fact that hormones combine with specific enzymes to be transported.
    D. The ability of hormones to have specific effects in very small quantities.
    E. The specific organ responsible for hormone production.

78. The bone in the upper leg (thigh) is the
    A. Fibula.
    B. Talus.
    C. Femur.
    D. Tibia.
    E. Patella.

79. Which of these muscles is innervated by nerve root C7?
    A. Biceps
    B. Triceps
    C. Subscapular
    D. Rhomboid
    E. Deep flexors of the fingers

80. Growth hormone
    A. Promotes increase in size of only specific tissue.
    B. Is secreted only until puberty is reached.
    C. Is secreted by the anterior pituitary.
    D. Is secreted by the posterior pituitary.
    E. Increases the size of individual tissues until puberty is reached.

81. The hypothalamo-hypophysial portal system
    A. Transports chemical messengers from the hypothalamus to the posterior pituitary.
    B. Carries nerve impulses from the hypothalamus to the pituitary.
    C. Carries release factors from the hypothalamus to the adenohypophysis.
    D. Facilitates the breakdown of chemicals into specific enzymes used by the hypothalamus.
    E. None of the above.

82. Elasticity of large circulatory vessels is important in
    A. Maintaining blood pressure and flow during heart relaxation.
    B. Determining degree of peripheral resistance.
    C. Determining distribution of blood volume to major areas of the body.
    D. Autoregulation of blood flow.
    E. Maintaining heart rhythm.

83. Antidiuretic hormone
    A. Is secreted by the kidneys.
    B. Is secreted by the neurohypophysis.
    C. Promotes water loss through the kidneys.
    D. Promotes sodium retention through the kidneys.
    E. Is secreted by the hypothalamus.

84. You have been told that you should gain weight. To do so, you should start to
    A. Become more active in order to greatly increase your appetite.
    B. Eat foods that are high in bulk.
    C. Eat foods that are low in bulk but high in calories.
    D. Try to sleep less.
    E. Exercise more.

85. Two activities of the menstrual cycle that occur simultaneously are
    A. Uterine proliferation and menstrual flow.
    B. Uterine proliferation and ovulation.
    C. Uterine proliferation and follicle development.
    D. Uterine proliferation and implantation.
    E. Uterine implantation and contraction.

86. The primary function of the spleen is to

    _____.

    A. Filter poisons out of the blood and produce mediators for blood clotting
    B. Filter toxins from the blood and regulate the body's electrolyte level
    C. Produce and destroy blood cells during systemic infection
    D. Provide a major source of estrogen and progesterone for the human body
    E. Store vitamins A, E, and K and produce vitamin D

87. Movement of the arms during the first count of a jumping jack relates to which motion?
    A. Adduction
    B. Abduction
    C. Flexion
    D. Extension
    E. Circumduction

88. Hypopolarized membranes
    A. Conduct action potentials with less ease than do normally polarized membranes.
    B. Conduct action potentials with less stimulation than do normally polarized membranes.
    C. Have a threshold point that is lower than normal.
    D. Conduct action potentials with greater stimulation than do hyperpolarized membranes.

    E. Conduct action potentials equivalent to those of normally polarized membranes.

89. Aspirin is effective in
    A. Curing the cause of headaches.
    B. Combating the cold virus.
    C. Reducing fever.
    D. Relieving stomach upset.
    E. Preventing pregnancy.

90. A sexually transmitted disease is usually contracted during
    A. Hand contact with an infected person.
    B. Mouth contact with an infected person.
    C. Sexual contact with an infected person.
    D. Conversation with an infected person.
    E. Genital contact with an infected toilet.

91. Immunization against the protein release factors that control the secretion of the gonadotropins is a/an
    A. Current contraceptive measure.
    B. New possibility for birth control.
    C. Postcoital contraceptive measure.
    D. Modern method of reconciling incompatible rhesus (Rh) blood factors.
    E. Ineffective method of birth control currently prohibited in the United States.

92. The muscular system is used for which of the following functions?
    A. Movement
    B. Signaling and integration
    C. Gas exchange
    D. Transportation of oxygen and cell nutrients
    E. Transportation of carbon dioxide and waste products

93. The myometrium is
    A. The site of fertilization.
    B. A muscle layer.
    C. The site of implantation.
    D. The major source of progesterone.
    E. An estrogen-rich layer of tissue beneath the endometrium.

94. Calcium, phosphorus, and iron are examples of
    A. Fats.
    B. Oils.
    C. Carbohydrates.
    D. Minerals.
    E. Vitamins.

95. The major source of gonadotrophic hormones is the
    A. Anterior pituitary.
    B. Posterior pituitary.
    C. Hypothalmus.
    D. Gonads (ovaries and testes).
    E. Endometrium.

96. An athlete gets hit in the right cheek with a baseball. He is unable to smile on that side of his face. What nerve do you suspect is involved?
    A. Trigeminal
    B. Oculomotor
    C. Facial
    D. Hypoglossal
    E. Optic

97. The male counterpart(s) of the fallopian tubes is(are) the
    A. Vas deferens.
    B. Seminal vesicles.
    C. Bulbourethral glands.
    D. Corpora lutea.
    E. Testicles.

98. Trapping of energy by carrier molecules involves
    A. Glycolysis.
    B. The Krebs cycle.
    C. The electron transport chain.
    D. Glycogen formation.
    E. Enzymatic release.

99. Which of the following hormones best illustrates the target organ specificity concept?
    A. Growth hormone
    B. Thyroid-stimulating hormone
    C. Estrogen
    D. Insulin
    E. Luteinizing hormone

100. Cranial nerve X is named the
    A. Trigeminal.
    B. Vagus.
    C. Abducent.
    D. Olfactory.
    E. Facial.

101. The substance that can be converted to vitamin A in the human body is
    A. Tryptophan.
    B. Glucose.
    C. Vitamin D.
    D. Carotene.
    E. Vitamin A.

102. Progesterone and estrogen act together on the fully developed endometrium on the menstrual cycle's
    A. 1st day.
    B. 4th day.
    C. 18th day.
    D. 25th day.
    E. 35th day.

103. Forward movement of the arm during the forehand drive in tennis involves which of the following motions?
    A. Abduction.
    B. Adduction.
    C. Horizontal abduction.
    D. Horizontal adduction.
    E. Vertical adduction.

104. Which contraception method prevents ovulation?
    A. Foam
    B. Diaphragm
    C. Oral contraceptive
    D. Rhythm method
    E. Intrauterine device

105. Which contraception method prevents implantation?
    A. Foam
    B. Diaphragm
    C. Oral contraceptive
    D. Rhythm method
    E. Intrauterine device

106. Which contraception method destroys sperm?
    A. Foam
    B. Diaphragm
    C. Oral contraceptive
    D. Rhythm method
    E. Intrauterine device

107. Which contraception method prevents sperm/ova contact?
    A. Foam
    B. Diaphragm
    C. Oral contraceptive
    D. Rhythm method
    E. Intrauterine device

108. The distal row of carpal bones from radius to ulna consists of
    A. Scaphoid, lunate, triquetral, pisiform.
    B. Trapezoid, trapezium, lunate, scaphoid.
    C. Scaphoid, capitate, trapezoid, hamate.
    D. Trapezium, trapezoid, triquetral, pisiform.
    E. Trapezium, trapezoid, capitate, hamate.

109. What is the common name for myositis ossificans of the biceps?
    A. Burner/stinger
    B. Blocker's exostosis
    C. Axillary patch
    D. Tennis elbow
    E. Joint mice

110. Diuresis refers to
    A. Na^+ loss at the kidney.
    B. Water loss at the kidney.
    C. Antidiuretic hormone (ADH) release at the pituitary.
    D. Aldosterone release at the adrenal cortex.
    E. Increased ADH.

111. Reflexes that are typically protective in nature and that are usually initiated by pain are termed
    A. Flexor reflexes.
    B. Extensor reflexes.
    C. Inhibitory reflexes.
    D. Patellar reflexes.
    E. Protective reflexes.

112. Which is the function of the nervous system?
    A. Providing movement
    B. Signaling and integration
    C. Providing gas exchange
    D. Transportation of oxygen and cell nutrients
    E. Transportation of carbon dioxide and waste products

113. Saltatory conduction refers to the
    A. Flow of electrical activity across cell membranes because of the presence of electrolytes such as Na^+ and Cl^-.
    B. Jumping movement of nerve impulses from node to node along myelinated axons and dendrites.
    C. Events at the synapse that cause the electrical activity to flow from one neuron to the next.
    D. Activity of the receptor that sets up action potentials in the sensory neurons supplying the receptors.

    E. Electrical activity generated when electrolytes cross the blood-brain barrier.

114. Frequency coding in action potentials provide a mechanism for
    A. Depolarizing receptors.
    B. Keeping the body constantly informed of internal conditions.
    C. Relating different stimulus intensities to the central nervous system.
    D. Explaining adaptation of neurons.
    E. Repolarizing neuron receptors.

115. Adaptation of receptors is best described as
    A. Receptor fatigue.
    B. Fewer action potentials per unit of time despite constant stimulus strength.
    C. The ability of receptors to give graded responses.
    D. The ability of receptors to summate.
    E. The ability of receptors to adapt to any environment.

116. Action potentials
    A. Result from membrane permeability changes.
    B. Are graded in magnitude according to the receptor.
    C. Are localized fluctuations of the membrane potential.
    D. Are graded in magnitude according to membrane potential.
    E. Result from changes in the receptor permeability.

117. Centers for regulation of vital functions such as respiration and heart rate are located in the
    A. Pons.
    B. Medulla.
    C. Cerebellum.
    D. Spinal cord.
    E. Frontal lobe.

118. Which of the following functional areas of the cerebral cortex deals with complex problems and abstract thought?
    A. Parietal lobe
    B. Temporal lobe
    C. Frontal lobe
    D. Occipital lobe
    E. Medulla

119. Latissimus dorsi, teres major, greater pectoral, and subscapular muscles all perform what motion?
    A. Adduction, scapular
    B. Abduction, scapular
    C. Internal rotation
    D. External rotation
    E. Stabilization

120. The articulation of first metacarpal with the carpal bone is a
    A. Biaxial joint.
    B. Diarthrodial joint.
    C. Saddle joint.
    D. Condyloid joint.
    E. Suture joint.

121. What is an action potential?
    A. A series of events marked by change in polarization of the cell membrane
    B. The transmission of a nerve impulse across a synapse
    C. The recovery of the nerve following passage of an impulse
    D. The action of the sodium pump
    E. The summation of acetylcholine

122. A woman whose daily caloric intake was 1700 cal and whose energy expenditure was 1900 kcal would have observed her weight to change

    by approximately _____ pounds by the end of 1 year.
    A. 21
    B. 19
    C. 10
    D. 25
    E. 15

123. Nodes of Ranvier are most closely associated with
    A. Secretion of adrenalin.
    B. Saltatory conduction of nerve impulses.
    C. Unmyelinated neurons.
    D. Integrative functions of the nervous system.
    E. Demyelinated nerve endings.

124. Which of the following holds one muscular attachment area in place?
    A. Stabilizer
    B. Mover
    C. Supporting muscles

    D. Neutralizer
    E. Antagonists

125. Angle of bend at the knee or elbow joint relates to a/an
    A. Chemoreceptor.
    B. Electromagnetic receptor.
    C. Thermoreceptor.
    D. Mechanoreceptor.
    E. Sensitoreceptor.

126. Darkness versus bright sunlight relates to a/an
    A. Chemoreceptor.
    B. Electromagnetic receptor.
    C. Thermoreceptor.
    D. Mechanoreceptor.
    E. Sensitoreceptor.

127. Sound and waves striking the eardrum relates to a/an
    A. Chemoreceptor.
    B. Electromagnetic receptor.
    C. Thermoreceptor.
    D. Mechanoreceptor.
    E. Sensitoreceptor.

128. Electrical summation with high-frequency stimulation is in the
    A. Receptor region.
    B. Conductile region.
    C. Transmissional region.
    D. Contractile region.
    E. Motor region.

129. The term *posterior* refers to which of the following?
    A. Toward the head
    B. Toward the midline of the body
    C. Toward the trunk
    D. Back portion of the body
    E. Away from the trunk

130. Antigen-antibody reactions can lead to renal failure as
    A. Chronic renal insufficiency.
    B. Tubular abnormalities.
    C. The nephrotic syndrome.
    D. Acute glomerular nephritis.
    E. The overflow phenomena.

131. Strength of stimulus is coded as a frequency of action potentials in the
    A. Receptor region.
    B. Conductile region.
    C. Transmissional region.
    D. Contractile region.
    E. Motor region.

132. The form in which fats principally occur in foods is as
    A. Triglycerides.
    B. Sterols.
    C. Phospholipids.
    D. Glycerols.
    E. Fatty acids.

133. An active nerve would show the first sign of fatigue in the
    A. Receptor region.
    B. Conductile region.
    C. Transmissional region.
    D. Contractile region.
    E. Motor region.

134. Fluorine is necessary in the body for
    A. Strength of bones and teeth.
    B. Production of thyroid hormone.
    C. Prevention of anemia.
    D. Metabolism of glucose.
    E. Breakdown of amino acids.

135. The term *anterior* refers to which of the following?
    A. Toward the feet
    B. Away from the midline of the body
    C. Away from the trunk
    D. Front portion of the body
    E. Back portion of the body

136. The Weber-Fechner Law relates to the
    A. Receptor region.
    B. Conductile region.
    C. Transmissional region.
    D. Contractile region.
    E. Motor region.

137. Troponin and tropomyosin are
    A. Contractile proteins.
    B. Inhibitory proteins.
    C. Antigenic proteins.
    D. Conductive proteins.
    E. Reactive proteins.

138. Tight junctions are
    A. Points of nutrient exchange between skeletal muscle cells.
    B. Waves of contractions moving through groups of smooth muscle cells.
    C. Points of electrical contact between smooth muscle cells.
    D. Sites where transmitter agents can stimulate smooth muscle cells.
    E. Points of neuromuscular crossbridges between skeletal and smooth muscle cells.

139. A diet low in carbohydrates but with enough protein and fat to meet theoretical energy needs may produce which of the following effects?
    A. Positive nitrogen balance
    B. Buildup of ketones in the body
    C. Increased conversion of fatty acids to glucose
    D. Negative nitrogen balance
    E. Increased conversion of amino acids to proteins

140. The function of the ureters is
    A. Excretion of urine.
    B. Collection of urine.
    C. Final pathway for elimination.
    D. Collection of urine and drainage into bladder.
    E. Absorption of water before urination.

141. Within certain limits, changes in strength of stimulation applied to a muscle result in a graded contractile response of the muscle because
    A. It is necessary for a muscle to contract smoothly.
    B. Individual fibers have different thresholds.
    C. This tends to retard the onset of fatigue.
    D. Every muscle has a predetermined contractile response.
    E. Certain fibers respond differently according to changes in muscle stimulation.

142. The dietary need for which one of the following vitamins is influenced by the presence of tryptophan in the diet?
    A. Thiamine
    B. Pantothenic acid
    C. Niacin
    D. Biotin
    E. Riboflavin

143. The trapezius muscle and the levator muscle of the scapula perform what motion?
    A. Elevation
    B. Depression
    C. Downward rotation
    D. Upward rotation
    E. Stabilization

144. Wave summation differs from tetany chiefly by an increase of
    A. Fatigue.
    B. Stimulus frequency.
    C. Stimulus intensity.
    D. Drum speed.
    E. Stimulus duration.

145. Myosin crossbridges contain active sites for which of the following?
    A. Ca^{++} and adenosine triphosphate (ATP)
    B. Troponin-tropomyosin and ATP
    C. Actin and ATP
    D. Only ATP
    E. Ca^{++} and troponin-tropomyosin

146. The largest structural feature of muscle is
    A. Myofilament.
    B. Myofibril.
    C. Sarcomere.
    D. Crossbridge.
    E. Z line.

147. The mechanical activity of smooth muscle may be described as
    A. Myogenic.
    B. Peristalsis.
    C. Slow fatigue.
    D. Spontaneous.
    E. Contraction.

148. Activation of glucose involves
    A. Glycolysis.
    B. The Krebs cycle.
    C. The electron transport chain.
    D. Glycogen formation.
    E. Enzymatic release.

149. Taping joints has
    A. Been proven to be the only effective way to protect them against injury.
    B. Been used with little knowledge of its effectiveness.
    C. Been shown to be a must in all postsurgical situations.
    D. Demonstrated little effectiveness in athletics.
    E. Been proven to give athletes a false sense of security.

150. Production of lactic acid involves
    A. Glycolysis.
    B. The Krebs cycle.
    C. The electron transport chain.
    D. Glycogen formation.
    E. Enzymatic release.

151. Blood returns to the heart from the body via the
    A. Aortic arch.
    B. Pulmonary artery.
    C. Pulmonary vein.
    D. Superior and inferior vena cava.
    E. Left ascending coronary artery.

152. Biochemical reactions run the fastest during periods of high-energy demand involving
    A. Glycolysis.
    B. The Krebs cycle.
    C. The electron transport chain.
    D. Glycogen formation.
    E. Enzymatic release.

153. The function of the pancreas is
    A. Storage of bile and vitamins A, B, and D.
    B. Secretion of insulin, hormone production for carbohydrate metabolism, and production of enzymes.
    C. Production of enzymes, storage of bile, and secretion of insulin.
    D. Storage of glucose and vitamins A, B, and E.
    E. Absorption of water.

154. Muscle that is autorhythmic and has a low length-tension relation is
    A. Smooth muscle.
    B. Skeletal muscle.
    C. Cardiac muscle.
    D. Sensitive muscle.
    E. Abdominal muscle.

155. Jaundice
    A. Results from oversecretion of bile into the small intestine.
    B. Results from the precipitation of cholesterol into gallstones that occlude the bile duct.

C. Results from poor breakdown of fats in the diet.

D. Is a term used to note the presence of undigested fat in the feces.

E. Results from the malabsorption of protein in the diet.

156. Movement along the long axis of the humerus while pitching a baseball involves which of the following motions?
    A. Flexion
    B. Pronation
    C. Circumduction
    D. Rotation
    E. Abduction

157. Sodium bicarbonate
    A. Is an enzyme from the pancreas.
    B. Neutralizes acidity in the stomach.
    C. Is a substance that is regulated by the hormone secretin.
    D. Absorbs acid in the body, thereby neutralizing the pH of the blood.
    E. Is an enzyme from the gallbladder.

158. Hitting a tennis ball at the top of the arc is desirable because of
    A. Summation of forces.
    B. Trading distances for forces.
    C. Angular and linear velocity change with length of lever.
    D. Greatest linear velocity at perpendicular to axis of rotation.
    E. Moment of force.

159. The usual consequence of a decreased protein concentration in the blood is
    A. Edema.
    B. Alkalosis.
    C. Acidosis.
    D. Phagocytosis.
    E. Anorexia.

160. Two substances that are secreted into the kidney tubules include
    A. Na^+ and K^+.
    B. Na^+ and H^+.
    C. H^+ and K^+.
    D. H^+ and Cl^-.
    E. Na^+ and Cl^-.

161. The miscellaneous group represented in the daily food plan usually supplies significant amounts of which nutrients?
    A. Low-quality protein
    B. High-quality protein
    C. Vitamins and minerals
    D. Carbohydrate and fat
    E. Protein and fat

162. The forearm flexor muscles during a push-up are
    A. Prime movers.
    B. Antagonists.
    C. Synergists.
    D. Stabilizers.
    E. Neutralizers.

163. Which of the statements below is not a function of hydrochloric acid (HCl)?
    A. Activates enzymes secreted in the stomach
    B. Kills bacteria that may enter the digestive tube along with the food
    C. Denatures proteins and breaks intramolecular bonds
    D. Enhances the activity of salivary amylase
    E. Neutralizes the pH of acids found in the stomach

164. Injecting urea into the bloodstream would cause
    A. Increased glomerular filtration.
    B. Increased reabsorption of water.
    C. Increased secretion of K^+.
    D. Increased urine volume.
    E. Decreased reabsorption of water causing a decrease in urine volume.

165. Reabsorption of electrolytes and water by the kidney is most dependent on
    A. Facilitated diffusion.
    B. Pinocytosis.
    C. Active transport.
    D. Osmosis.
    E. Passive transport.

166. What substance is a product of protein digestion?
    A. Amino acid
    B. Ammonia
    C. Pyruvic acid
    D. Urea
    E. Glucose

167. The glenohumeral joint allows for how many degrees of freedom?
    A. One
    B. Two
    C. Three
    D. Four
    E. Five

168. During protein digestion
    A. Water molecules are removed from peptide bonds, thereby splitting the amino acids apart.
    B. Pepsin is inhibited by the high acidity of the stomach.
    C. Hydrochloric acid (HCl) secretion is decreased because of the action of pancreatic amylase.
    D. HCl secretion is increased because of the hormone gastrin.
    E. Sodium bicarbonate secretion is increased because of the acidity in the stomach.

169. In what way does the interior surface of the membrane of a nonconducting neuron differ from the external surface?
    A. It is negatively charged and contains less sodium.
    B. It is positively charged and contains less sodium.
    C. It is negatively charged and contains more sodium.
    D. It is positively charged and contains more sodium.
    E. It may be negatively or positively charged depending on the amount of sodium.

170. The radius in flexion of the forearm is an example of a
    A. First-class lever.
    B. Second-class lever.
    C. Third-class lever.
    D. Fourth-class lever.
    E. Fifth-class lever.

171. Active transport of monosaccharides across the intestinal wall relates to which function?
    A. Digestion
    B. Secretion
    C. Motility
    D. Absorption
    E. Elimination

172. The fat-soluble vitamins
    A. Are less stable than the water-soluble vitamins are.
    B. Require bile for absorption.
    C. Are the B vitamins and vitamin C.
    D. Are minimally stored in the body; therefore deficiency symptoms often develop rapidly.
    E. Are usually constituents of coenzymes.

173. The action of carboxypeptidase in the small intestine relates to which function?
    A. Digestion
    B. Secretion
    C. Motility
    D. Absorption
    E. Elimination

174. Which ligaments make up the lateral ligaments of the elbow?
    A. Radial collateral ligament, lateral ulnar collateral ligament, anterior oblique band, posterior oblique band
    B. Transverse oblique band, annular ligament, accessory collateral ligament, radial collateral ligament
    C. Radial collateral ligament, lateral ulnar collateral ligament, accessory collateral ligament, anterior oblique band
    D. Anterior oblique band, posterior oblique band, transverse oblique band, annular ligament
    E. Annular ligament, accessory collateral ligament, radial collateral ligament, lateral ulnar collateral ligament

175. Production of bicarbonate from the pancreas relates to which function?
    A. Digestion
    B. Secretion
    C. Motility
    D. Absorption
    E. Elimination

176. Emulsification relates to which function?
    A. Digestion
    B. Secretion
    C. Motility
    D. Absorption
    E. Elimination

177. Formation of chylomicrons relates to which function?
    A. Digestion
    B. Secretion
    C. Motility
    D. Absorption
    E. Elimination

178. The propulsive phase of the femur during running involves which of the following motions?
    A. Flexion
    B. Extension
    C. Abduction
    D. Adduction
    E. Circumduction

179. The action of pancreozymin or trypsin relates to which function?
    A. Digestion
    B. Secretion
    C. Motility
    D. Absorption
    E. Elimination

180. Movement of the upper arm during a push-up relates to what motion?
    A. Horizontal abduction
    B. Horizontal adduction
    C. Flexion
    D. Extension
    E. Vertical abduction

181. The process by which leukocytes squeeze through pores in the capillary wall is termed
    A. Diapedesis.
    B. Leukotaxis.
    C. Phagocytosis.
    D. Pinocytosis.
    E. Chemotaxis.

182. The most significant value of macrophages is their ability to
    A. Quickly counteract bacterial invasion.
    B. Reach injured areas quickly.
    C. Engulf large quantities of bacteria.
    D. Dissolve in large quantities of tissue.
    E. Prevent bacterial invasion.

183. Blood flow in the heart and brain is regulated by localized needs. This method of regulation is termed
    A. Negative feedback.
    B. Chemoreceptor control.
    C. Autoregulation.
    D. Hyperventilation.
    E. Hypoventilation.

184. The term *lateral* refers to which of the following?
    A. Toward the feet
    B. Away from the midline of the body
    C. Away from the trunk
    D. Front portion of the body
    E. Back portion of the body

185. Failure of the left ventricle would most likely cause
    A. Decreased hematocrit.
    B. Nutritional edema.
    C. Increased secretion of heparin.
    D. Pulmonary edema.
    E. Death.

186. What is the most important stabilizing structure on the lateral elbow?
    A. Radial collateral ligament.
    B. Ulnar collateral ligament.
    C. Accessory lateral collateral ligament.
    D. Lateral ulnar collateral ligament.
    E. Annular ligament.

187. Normal stroke volume of the heart is
    A. 120 mL/min.
    B. 70 mL/beat.
    C. 45 mL/beat.
    D. 5000 mL/min.
    E. 62 mL/h.

188. The glenohumeral joint is in a closed-packed position when
    A. The humerus is in anatomic position.
    B. The humerus is abducted to 90 degrees and externally rotated.
    C. The humerus is abducted to 90 degrees and internally rotated.
    D. The humerus is flexed to 180 degrees and externally rotated.
    E. The humerus is flexed to 180 degrees and internally rotated.

189. Increases in cardiac output are usually obtained through increases in
    A. Stroke volume.
    B. Heart rate.
    C. Venous return.
    D. Blood pressure.
    E. Respiratory rate.

190. The most potent agent regulating respiration is
    A. Oxygen concentration of the blood
    B. Carbon dioxide levels at the respiratory center.
    C. Lactic acid levels in the blood.
    D. Glucose levels in the blood.
    E. Oxygen levels in the hypothalamus.

191. The corpus luteum secretes
    A. Only estrogen.
    B. Only progesterone.
    C. Both estrogen and progesterone.
    D. Neither estrogen nor progesterone.
    E. A follicle-stimulating hormone.

192. Subject A has a respiratory rate of 14 respirations per minute and a tidal volume of 475 ml per breath. Assuming the normal dead space volume, subject A's alveolar ventilation rate would be
    A. 4550 mL/min.
    B. 6550 mL/min.
    C. 1500 mL/min.
    D. 2100 mL/min.
    E. 5210 mL/min.

193. During inhalation
    A. Atmospheric pressure is lower than intrapleural pressure.
    B. Intra-alveolar pressure is lower than intrapleural pressure.
    C. Intra-alveolar pressure is lower than atmospheric pressure.
    D. Intra-alveolar pressure is higher than atmospheric pressure.
    E. Intrapleual pressure is higher than atmospheric pressure.

194. Negative pressure in the respiratory system is normally always found in the
    A. Alveoli.
    B. Bronchi.
    C. Intrapleural space.
    D. Atmosphere.
    E. Blood.

195. Which of these muscles is not an internal rotator at the shoulder?
    A. Infraspinous
    B. Teres major
    C. Latissimus dorsi
    D. Greater pectoral
    E. Subscapular

196. An electrocardiogram is a record of
    A. Impulse conduction through the heart.
    B. The rate and strength of heart contractions.
    C. The vibrations produced by heart valves.
    D. The volume of blood flowing through coronary arteries.
    E. The sounds the heart makes as the valves open and close.

197. Which of the following would be the most effective way to protect an anterior thigh contusion on a basketball player?
    A. A neoprene sleeve
    B. A doughnut pad with a thermoplastic dome
    C. A ½-inch solid closed cell pad
    D. A compression elastic wrap
    E. A hip spica dressing

198. Which of the following is not a precursor to myositis ossificans?
    A. Genetic formation of abnormal tissue
    B. Massage to a sore muscle in late rehabilitation
    C. Bloodborne disease
    D. Trauma
    E. Neurological disease

199. Over-the-counter weight reduction pills contain diuretics that produce weight loss by
    A. Decreasing appetite.
    B. Eliminating carbohydrates from the diet.
    C. Changing basic patterns of eating.
    D. Causing the kidneys to excrete more water.
    E. Sparing carbohydrates.

200. Which of the following structures is not considered dead space in the human respiratory system?
    A. Nasal passages
    B. Trachea
    C. Bronchi
    D. Alveoli
    E. Pharnyx

201. An abnormally long patellar tendon can lead to the condition of
    A. Patella alta.
    B. Patella baja.
    C. Squinting patella.
    D. "Frog-eyed" patella.
    E. Camel sign.

202. Use of oxygen involves
    A. Glycolysis.
    B. The Krebs cycle.
    C. The electron transport chain.
    D. Glycogen formation.
    E. Enzymatic release.

203. Normal dead space volume in the human respiratory system is
    A. 15 mL.
    B. 500 mL.
    C. 5000 mL.
    D. 150 mL.
    E. 550 mL.

204. Which of the following is not the effect of nicotine on the cardiovascular system?
    A. Vasoconstriction
    B. Slower heart rate
    C. Skipping of heartbeats
    D. Erratic heart rhythm
    E. Higher heart rate

205. The upper limit of safety for cholesterol concentration in the blood is
    A. 150 mg%.
    B. 250 mg%.
    C. 350 mg%.
    D. 500 mg%.
    E. 400 mg%.

206. Atherosclerosis is
    A. A disease process involving inflammation of the kidneys.
    B. A disease process that begins at middle age and causes death mostly in old age.
    C. Commonly referred to as a disease of starvation.
    D. A disease process that causes fatty deposits to build up on the inner walls of coronary arteries.
    E. A disease process that causes the coronary arteries to dilate, allowing more blood flow to the heart.

207. What nerve travels with the superficial flexor muscle of the fingers?
    A. Musculocutaneous nerve
    B. Radial nerve
    C. Median nerve
    D. Ulnar nerve
    E. Axillary nerve

208. Diabetic coma is a result of
    A. Depressed fat metabolism that cannot supply energy when glucose is scarce.
    B. The accumulation of insulin in the bloodstream without carbohydrate on which it can act.
    C. The increased concentration of H^+ in the blood arising from ketone bodies.
    D. Poor circulation to the brain because of the buildup of fatty deposits (arteriosclerosis) in the arterial tree.
    E. Oversecretion of insulin.

209. Calculate the energy value of this meal:

FOOD	PROTEIN	FAT	CHO
One hamburger	17 g	22 g	40 g
One large cola			25 g
One order French fries	4 g	14 g	40 g

The number of calories from protein were
    A. 21.
    B. 84.
    C. 88.
    D. 185.
    E. 189.

210. The hormone necessary for milk release during nursing is
  A. Oxytocin.
  B. Antidiuretic hormone.
  C. Progesterone.
  D. Estrogen.
  E. Follicle-stimulating hormone.

211. Based on what you know about fat metabolism, you would advise the person wanting to lose weight by exercising to
  A. Work with average effort for long periods of time.
  B. Work intensely for short periods with rest between periods.
  C. Work for prolonged periods with a slight oxygen debt.
  D. Carbohydrate load the muscles before each workout.
  E. Consume a protein-rich diet before exercise.

212. Which of the following organizational levels would provide the best source of information about electron transport activities when studying metabolism?
  A. A cellular homogenate
  B. An isolated, perfused liver
  C. The microsomal fraction
  D. The soluble fraction
  E. The mitochondrial fraction

213. What percentage of a given amount of lactic acid must be oxidized to carbon dioxide and water to provide the energy to generate glucose from the remaining lactic acid?
  A. 15%
  B. 30%
  C. 45%
  D. 60%
  E. 25%

214. Vitamin deficiencies exert their effects in metabolic activities because of their role as
  A. Stimulators of enzyme activity.
  B. Regulators of transport activities at the cell membrane.
  C. Necessary cofactors for enzyme activity such as nicotinamide adenine dinucleotide (NAD), nicotinamide adenine dinucleotide phosphate (NADP), or flavin adenine dinucleotide (FAD).

  D. Activators of acetylcoenzyme A.
  E. Neutralizers of cellular activity.

215. Essential amino acids must be obtained in the diet because
  A. Cells cannot transaminate all of the appropriate compounds to produce all the needed amino acids.
  B. Cells do not have access to hydroxyl and sulfur groups necessary for some amino acids.
  C. Cells cannot construct the correct carbon skeleton to which the appropriate functional groups could be added.
  D. Certain biochemical reactions are irreversible.
  E. Cell death can occur within 48 hours if the proper amino acids are not supplied by the diet.

216. Ovulation occurs as the result of
  A. Estrogen secretion during the follicular phase.
  B. The sharp rise in luteinizing hormone secretion around the 13th and 14th days of the female menstrual cycle.
  C. The rise in progesterone levels.
  D. Oxytoxin release from the posterior pituitary.
  E. The decline in progesterone levels around the 7th and 8th days of the female menstrual cycle.

217. The term *proximal* refers to which of the following?
  A. Toward the head
  B. Toward the midline of the body
  C. Toward the trunk
  D. Back portion of the body
  E. Away from the midline of the body

218. Operating a pair of pliers would be an example of a
  A. First-class lever.
  B. Second-class lever.
  C. Third-class lever.
  D. Fourth-class lever.
  E. Fifth-class lever.

219. The mobile wad of three consists of which three muscles?
   A. Ulnar extensor of the wrist, short radial extensor of the wrist, long radial extensor of the wrist.
   B. Ulnar flexor of the wrist, radial flexor of the wrist, long palmar.
   C. Short radial extensor of the wrist, long radial extensor of the wrist, brachioradial.
   D. Radial flexor of the wrist, round pronator, long palmar.
   E. Brachioradial, brachial, biceps of the arm.

220. Electrochemical equilibrium is a balance of
   A. Diffusion force and membrane polarity.
   B. Passive transport and active transport.
   C. Negative charge inside and positive charge outside.
   D. Na^+ influx and K^+ efflux.
   E. Osmosis and cellular polarity.

221. The tendon distal to the patella is called the
   A. Quadriceps tendon.
   B. Patellar tendon.
   C. Bicipital tendon.
   D. Tibial tendon.
   E. Femoral tendon.

222. The type of material capable of absorbing force through deforming its shape and then quickly returning to its original form is
   A. High-density foam.
   B. Low-density foam.
   C. Moleskin.
   D. Felt.
   E. Thermomoldable plastic.

223. In the resting condition a potential exists across the nerve cell membrane. This potential is a result of
   A. The negatively charged protein drawing Na^+ into the cell.
   B. The relatively high steady-state flux of K^+ back and forth across the membrane.
   C. The difference in the magnitude of Na^+ and K^+ concentration gradients.
   D. The Cl^- equilibrium potential.
   E. The polarity disparity between Na^+ and Cl^-.

224. The tennis serve (movement of the criterion arm) is done in which plane?
   A. Frontal
   B. Transverse
   C. Sagittal
   D. Medial
   E. Lateral

225. Sensory receptors that obey the Weber-Fechner Laws
   A. Can convert a large range of stimulus strengths into meaningful action potential frequencies.
   B. Only detect stimuli in a narrow range of stimulus intensity.
   C. Seldom undergo adaptation.
   D. Conduct action potentials of the same magnitude once threshold has been reached.
   E. Detect stimuli of a greater stimulus intensity.

226. While you are opening a door, the door is a
   A. First-class lever.
   B. Second-class lever.
   C. Third-class lever.
   D. Fourth-class lever.
   E. Fifth-class lever.

227. The inferior fibers of the trapezius and the latissimus dorsi muscles perform what motion?
   A. Flexion
   B. Extension
   C. Abduction, glenohumeral
   D. Adduction, glenohumeral
   E. Stabilization

228. The second messenger hypothesis suggests that
   A. Cyclic AMP stimulates receptor molecules at the surface of target cells.
   B. Adenylcyclase stimulates interior cell responses for particular hormones.
   C. Hormones combining with receptor molecules stimulate adenylcyclase, which increases cyclic AMP production.
   D. There are two messengers by which cyclic AMP is transported to target cells.
   E. Multiple enzymes contribute to cellular responses for specific hormones.

229. The renal fraction refers to the
   A. Amount of blood flowing through the capillary system of the kidneys.
   B. Total volume of blood pumped by the heart each minute that ends up in the renal circulation.
   C. Amount of blood filtered at the glomeruli of the kidneys.
   D. Amount of blood entering the renal artery divided by that which passes out the renal vein.
   E. Amount of blood leaving the renal vein as it is filtered at the glomeruli of the kidneys.

230. Which of the following is not associated with heart disease?
   A. High intake of animal fats
   B. Cigarette smoking
   C. Lack of exercise
   D. Vegetarian diet
   E. Stress

231. Reabsorption from the kidney tubule system depends most on
   A. Facilitated diffusion.
   B. Pinocytosis.
   C. Osmosis.
   D. Active transport.
   E. Passive transport.

232. Which part of the tooth is dead tissue?
   A. Dentin
   B. Enamel
   C. Pulp
   D. Gum
   E. Root

233. Osmotic diuresis results from
   A. Low antidiuretic hormone (ADH) output.
   B. The overflow phenomena.
   C. Reduced protein concentration in the blood.
   D. Kidney tubules that are insensitive to ADH.
   E. Increased protein concentration in the kidney tubules.

234. An easy way to spot an athlete with tight hamstrings is by
   A. Watching the way he or she walks.
   B. Checking back flexibility.
   C. Watching his or her sitting position when having ankles taped.
   D. Checking for gastrocnemius tightness.
   E. Watching the way he or she runs during warm-up exercises.

235. Basophils are important because
   A. They combat certain parasitic infections and allergic reactions.
   B. They are extremely mobile and respond quickly to invasion of microorganisms.
   C. They are extremely phagocytic.
   D. They release heparin into the bloodstream.
   E. They retain heparin.

236. To comply with current recommendations, the protein to fat to carbohydrate ratio should be
   A. 10:40:50.
   B. 10:50:40.
   C. 15:40:35.
   D. 15:30:55.
   E. 10:30:45.

237. During ventricular systole
   A. The second heart sound is heard.
   B. The aortic valves open.
   C. The atrioventricular valves open.
   D. The P wave could be recorded.
   E. A T wave could be recorded.

238. The term *superior* refers to which of the following?
   A. Toward the midline of the body
   B. Toward the head
   C. Toward the trunk
   D. Back portion of the body
   E. Front portion of the body

239. Negative feedback control is illustrated by decreased production of
   A. Testosterone as a result of low luteinizing hormone (LH) blood levels.
   B. LH as a result of low testosterone blood levels.
   C. LH as a result of high testosterone blood levels.
   D. LH because of inherent rhythmicity of specialized neurosecretory cells.
   E. Estrogen as a result of low testosterone and high LH blood levels.

240. Summation of ventricular contractile activity is prevented by the
    A. Compensory pause.
    B. Extrasystole.
    C. Absolute refractory period.
    D. Inherent sinoatrial (SA) rhythm.
    E. Diastolic phase.

241. The primary function of the diencephalon is to
    _____.
    A. Control the body's primary motor functions, both gross muscle contraction and coordination of the muscle contractions, in a specific sequence
    B. Act as a processing center for conscious and unconscious brain input
    C. Process sensory information such as temperature, pain, pressure, and proprioception
    D. Provide the functions necessary to maintain balance and coordination of the lower extremities
    E. Send efferent messages to the upper extremity

242. The most common condition leading to the onset of cardiac problems in middle-aged and older athletes is _____.
    A. Cystic fibrosis
    B. Marfan syndrome
    C. Cardiac arrhythmia
    D. Atherosclerosis
    E. Hypertrophic cardiomyopathy

243. Which of the following paths constitutes the normal route for conduction of electrical activity through the heart?
    A. Sinoatrial (SA) node to atrioventricular (AV) node to AV bundle to Purkinje fibers to ventricular musculature
    B. SA node to atrial musculature to AV node to AV bundle to bundle branches to ventricular musculature
    C. SA node to atrial musculature to AV node to AV bundle to bundle branches to Purkinje fibers to ventricular musculature
    D. SA node to AV node to AV bundle to bundle branches to Purkinje fibers
    E. SA node to AV bundle to atrial musculature to AV node to bundle branches to ventricular musculature to Purkinje fibers

244. What two muscles make up the hypothenar eminence?
    A. Superficial flexor and deep flexor muscles of the fingers
    B. Dorsal interosseous and palmar interosseous muscles
    C. Long abductor and short abductor of the thumb
    D. Abductor muscle and opposing muscle of the little finger
    E. Extensor muscle of the little finger and adductor muscle of the thumb

245. Which of the following are all disaccharides?
    A. Glucose, maltose, lactose
    B. Lactose, galactose, glucose
    C. Galactose, fructose, glucose
    D. Sucrose, fructose, maltose
    E. Maltose, lactose, sucrose

246. Air flow between the atmosphere and the alveoli during respiration is caused by
    A. Muscular contraction and relaxation of the lungs.
    B. Alternately rising and falling pressures in compartments surrounding the lungs.
    C. Diffusion gradients for individual gases between the atmosphere and lungs.
    D. Internal pressure gradients allowing air to flow in while atmospheric pressure is at its peak.
    E. External pressure gradients allowing the alveoli to open while air flows in.

247. What structure makes up the medial border of the femoral triangle?
    A. Long adductor muscle
    B. Inguinal ligament
    C. Sartorius muscle
    D. Gracilis muscle
    E. Quadrate muscle of the thigh

248. Which of the following directly causes a given motion?
    A. Stabilizer
    B. Prime mover
    C. Supporting muscles
    D. Neutralizer
    E. Antagonists

249. The advantages of combining dietary restriction with exercise in weight reduction include all except which one of the following?
    A. Allows a more liberal diet than is possible with a dietary restriction alone
    B. Improves distribution of nutrients to cells
    C. Decreases blood cholesterol
    D. Decreases the number of fat cells
    E. Improves use of fat for energy

250. Which of the following occurs approximately 7 days after fertilization?
    A. Dilation
    B. Ovulation
    C. Parturition
    D. Implantation
    E. Uterine instability

251. The type of lipid that serves as the precursor to the sex hormones and many other important molecules is
    A. Phospholipids.
    B. Cholesterol.
    C. Triglycerides.
    D. Bile salt.
    E. Cellulite.

252. The vasodilator theory of autoregulation suggests that
    A. Metabolic by-products increase blood flow by causing vasodilation in localized areas.
    B. Metabolic by-products enhance respiration to increase oxygen concentration in the blood.
    C. Metabolic by-products inhibit nerves supplying blood vessels leading to relaxation of smooth muscle producing vasodilation and increased blood flow.
    D. Local needs of oxygen determine the degree of vasotone and blood flow.
    E. Vasodilatation is caused by metabolic by-products decreasing blood flow to localized areas.

253. Which part of the tooth is alive and can be sensitive?
    A. Dentin
    B. Enamel
    C. Pulp
    D. Gum
    E. Root

254. Trophoblastic nutrition is a term to describe which of the following processes?
    A. The attachment of trophoblastic cell cords to the edges of the digested endometrium
    B. Breaking down and imbibing the secretory cells of the endometrium by the trophoblastic cells
    C. Development of the placenta and the extraembryonic membranes from the trophoblastic cell
    D. A method of sustaining the blastocyst that depends on estrogen secretion
    E. Nutrition essential to the formation of trophoblasts during the follicular phase of development

255. Conduction velocity in the atrioventricular (AV) bundle, bundle branches, and Purkinje fibers is much greater than it is in other nodal tissues. This is significant to heart function because
    A. The delay in conduction at the AV node must be made up for to keep the heart in time.
    B. It rapidly spreads electrical activity over the entire ventricular musculature to produce unified contraction, which results in greater pressure development.
    C. The inherently low discharge rates of these structures must be overcome.
    D. The ventricles have more mass, and velocity must be increased to complete all activities within 0.86 seconds.
    E. It can compensate for the low velocity produced by the ventricles.

256. Internal respiration consists of oxygen transport
    A. To cell level.
    B. To the blood.
    C. Across the cell membrane.
    D. From the atmosphere to the blood.
    E. From the cell to the atmosphere.

257. An essential amino acid found in dietary protein in a quantity that is less adequate than any other essential amino acid to meet the body's need is termed
    A. Indigestible.
    B. Low value.
    C. Reduced.
    D. Noncaloric.
    E. Limiting.

258. Ventilation of atmospheric air is produced by the
     A. Diaphragm drawing in air.
     B. Muscles drawing in air.
     C. Diaphragm and muscles drawing in air.
     D. Pressure differential between expanded chest and atmospheric air.
     E. Pressure differential between atmospheric air and contracted muscles drawing in air.

259. In the abdomen, the largest lymphatic organ(s) is(are) the _____.
     A. Liver
     B. Lungs
     C. Urinary bladder
     D. Spleen
     E. Kidneys

260. Movement of the arms during propulsive phase of the elementary backstroke relates to which motion?
     A. Adduction
     B. Abduction
     C. Flexion
     D. Extension
     E. Supination

261. The liver has which of the following functions?
     A. Secretion of insulin
     B. Absorption of water
     C. Storage of certain vitamins, detoxification, secretion of bile, and initiating metabolism
     D. Storage of bile
     E. Digestion with enzymes

262. The functions of the kidneys are
     A. Balance of water and acid-base and collection of urine.
     B. Balance of water and electrolytes and excretion of urine.
     C. Balance of water, electrolytes, and acid-base and excretion of urine.
     D. Balance of water, electrolytes, and acid-base and collection of urine.
     E. Balance of water and electrolytes and absorption of urine.

263. The normal distribution of electrolytes on the two sides of a neuron cell membrane is due to
     A. The concentration gradient.
     B. Passive transport.
     C. Active transport.
     D. Electrostatic repulsion.
     E. Osmosis.

264. The urethra has which of the following functions?
     A. Collection of urine
     B. Final passageway for elimination
     C. Reservoir for urine
     D. Helping to expel urine
     E. Accumulating electrolytes before urination

265. The primary function of the respiratory system is to
     A. Bring oxygen to the lungs.
     B. Get oxygen to the circulatory system.
     C. Get oxygen to cells.
     D. Transport oxygen and carbon dioxide to and from the cell.
     E. Bring carbon dioxide to the lungs.

266. The leukocyte can be best characterized by its
     A. Defense against microorganisms.
     B. Development of antibodies.
     C. Mobility through capillary wall.
     D. Storage of hemoglobin.
     E. Development of antigens.

267. Bile has which of the following functions?
     A. Emulsification of fat globules and dumping of fat metabolism end products into the lymphatic system
     B. Protein metabolism and filtration
     C. Protein metabolism and detoxification
     D. Fat metabolism and storage of vitamins A, B_{12}, and D
     E. Carbohydrate metabolism and protein metabolism

268. Menstrual flow ceases and the endometrium begins to repair itself and grow under the influence of rising blood estrogen concentration on the
     A. 1st day.
     B. 4th day.
     C. 18th day.
     D. 25th day.
     E. 35th day.

269. The appearance of striations on a skeletal muscle is due to the contrast of
    A. Z line and A band.
    B. A band and I band.
    C. A band and H zone.
    D. H zone and I band.
    E. A line and Z band.

270. The speed at which an impulse travels is due to
    A. Magnitude of the stimulus.
    B. Ability of the sodium pump.
    C. Permeability of the neuron membrane.
    D. Cross-sectional diameter and insulation.
    E. Duration of the stimulus.

271. If an athletic trainer is asked to select and fit a football helmet on a player's head, the primary criterion for selection of the helmet is that it
    A. Is equipped with the proper facemask for the player's position.
    B. Is approved by the National Operating Committee on Standards for Athletic Equipment (NOCSAE).
    C. Is cleaned and bacteria free.
    D. Is of the correct color to meet uniformity rules.
    E. Has jaw pads in place.

272. The correct organization of the body from its simplest unit to the most complex arrangement is
    A. Cell, organ, tissue, gland, system.
    B. Cell, gland, tissue, organ, system.
    C. Cell, tissue, gland, organ, system.
    D. Cell, gland, organ, tissue, system.
    E. Tissue, organ, gland, system.

273. The ventral cavity consists of
    A. Mediastinum and pelvic and pleural cavities.
    B. Thoracic and abdominal cavities.
    C. Abdominal and right and left pleural cavities.
    D. Right and left pleural cavities and abdominal cavity.
    E. Abdominal and mediastinal cavities.

274. Deposits of minerals in the kidneys, blood vessels, and other soft tissues in the body may be related to
    A. Excessive dietary vitamin A.
    B. Inadequate dietary vitamin D.
    C. Excessive dietary vitamin D.
    D. Excessive dietary vitamin K.
    E. Inadequate dietary vitamin K.

275. Connective tissue is
    A. Voluntary and fibrous.
    B. Reticular and voluntary.
    C. Reticular and collagenous.
    D. Voluntary and collagenous.
    E. Reticular and fibrous.

276. Which of the following is true regarding taping muscles?
    A. It reinforces muscular strength.
    B. It cannot be effectively accomplished.
    C. It will improve strength.
    D. It usually increases circulation.
    E. It should never be done.

277. The disintegration of the corpus luteum begins on the menstrual cycle's
    A. 1st day.
    B. 4th day.
    C. 18th day.
    D. 25th day.
    E. 35th day.

278. The skeletal system provides
    A. Homeostasis and waste removal.
    B. Locomotion and protection.
    C. Procreation.
    D. Preparation of food for absorption at cell level.
    E. Oxygenated blood to working muscles.

279. The force that the hands expend on the bat while swinging at the ball is
    A. Moment of force.
    B. Centrifugal force.
    C. Centripetal force.
    D. Summation of force.
    E. Distal force.

280. Blood contains
    A. Erythrocytes, leukocytes, platelets, and water.
    B. Erythrocytes, leukocytes, plasma, and solutes.
    C. Erythrocytes, leukocytes, platelets, and plasma.
    D. Erythrocytes, leukocytes, platelets, and solutes.
    E. Erythrocytes only.

281. Digestion of proteins begins in the
    A. Esophagus.
    B. Mouth.
    C. Stomach.
    D. Large intestine.
    E. Small intestine.

282. What three muscles insert on the pes anserinus?
    A. Semitendinous, semimembranous, sartorius
    B. Sartorius, gracilis, semimembranous
    C. Semitendinous, gracilis, sartorius
    D. Semitendinous, semimembranous, gracilis
    E. Semitendinous, gracilis, thigh biceps

283. Blood is pumped to the aortic arch by the
    A. Right auricle.
    B. Right ventricle.
    C. Left ventricle.
    D. Left auricle.
    E. Right atrium.

284. Distribution of oxygen and usable metabolic materials occurs through
    A. Arteries.
    B. Veins.
    C. Glands.
    D. Capillaries.
    E. Venules.

285. A suture articulation is
    A. Synarthrodial.
    B. Diarthrodial.
    C. Fibrous.
    D. Cartilaginous.
    E. Cellulous.

286. The elbow is an example of a/an
    A. Synarthrodial joint.
    B. Diarthrodial joint.
    C. Uniaxial joint.
    D. Hinge joint.
    E. Ball and socket joint.

287. The radioulnar articulation is a/an
    A. Diarthrodial joint.
    B. Uniaxial joint.
    C. Pivot joint.
    D. Biaxial joint.
    E. All of the above.

288. The most important factor in normal blood filtration at the kidneys is
    A. Blood protein concentration.
    B. Blood capillary pressure.
    C. Glomerular capillary permeability.
    D. Sympathetic constriction of renal arterioles.
    E. Parasympathetic dilatation of the glomerulus.

289. The difference between synarthrodial and diarthrodial articulations is that
    A. Synarthrodial articulations have joint capsules and synovial membrane and allow movement.
    B. Diarthrodial articulations have joint capsules and synovial membrane and allow movement.
    C. Allowance of movement is the only criterion.
    D. Synarthrodial articulations are cartilaginous.
    E. Synovial membranes are the only criteria.

290. The correct progression from the whole muscle to the sarcomere level is
    A. Fiber, fibrils, myofibrils.
    B. Fiber, myofibrils, fibrils.
    C. Fibrils, myofibrils, fibers.
    D. Myofibrils, fibrils, fiber.
    E. Fibrils, fibers, myofibrils.

291. An athlete should never blow his or her nose if suspected of having
    A. Corneal abrasion.
    B. Blow-out fracture.
    C. Ruptured globe.
    D. Conjunctivitis.
    E. Rhinorrhea.

292. A middle-distance runner suffers from exercise-induced asthma. Which of the following activities should be recommended to lessen the intensity of wheezing during workouts?
    A. Swimming
    B. Aerobic dancing
    C. Circuit weight training
    D. Bicycling
    E. Rope jumping

293. Which of the following is not characteristic of a vitamin?
   A. An organic compound
   B. A protein
   C. A substance that cannot be formed in the body
   D. A substance that is required in very small amounts
   E. A compound that in many instances increases the activity of an enzyme

294. A properly fitted mouth guard will assist in reducing all of the following injuries except
   A. Tooth fractures.
   B. Temporomandibular joint sprains.
   C. Fractured zygomatic bone.
   D. Intruded teeth.
   E. Cerebral concussions.

295. A significant indication of overtraining is
   A. Increased muscle tone.
   B. Increased flexibility.
   C. Increased urinary output.
   D. Increased performance.
   E. Increased pulse rate.

296. An athletic trainer should be able to discover disqualifying abnormalities and identify correctable or treatable physical conditions in an athlete by checking the athlete's
   A. Medical referral records.
   B. Athletic injury records.
   C. Preseason medical evaluation.
   D. Daily medical reports.
   E. Athletic injury reports.

297. During strenuous exercise, a diabetic's insulin requirement
   A. Is usually increased.
   B. Does not change.
   C. Depends on the athlete's weight.
   D. Is unpredictable.
   E. Is no longer needed.

298. When doing a push-up, the abdominal muscles act as
   A. Prime movers.
   B. Antagonists.
   C. Synergists.
   D. Stabilizers.
   E. Contractors.

299. Exercise-induced muscle soreness most commonly results from which type of muscle contraction?
   A. Concentric
   B. Eccentric
   C. Plyometric
   D. Isokinetic
   E. Isometric

300. Glycogen is
   A. An important blood protein.
   B. A disaccharide.
   C. A phospholipid.
   D. A polysaccharide.
   E. A monosaccharide.

301. Extrinsic factors influencing the onset of athletic injuries include all of the following except
   A. Gender.
   B. Environmental conditions.
   C. Type of playing surface.
   D. Type of protective headgear used.
   E. Time of day.

302. Illegal high school basketball equipment consists of
   A. A thigh pad with an unyielding surface.
   B. Pads objected to by the opposing coaches.
   C. An unpadded nose guard.
   D. Ensolite padding for a hand injury.
   E. Any unyielding material distal to the elbow.

303. In comparison with red (aerobic) muscle fibers, white (anaerobic) muscle fibers contain a higher level of
   A. Glycogen.
   B. Fat.
   C. Myoglobin.
   D. Protein.
   E. Hemoglobin.

304. A newborn baby lacks the ability to digest
   A. Lactose.
   B. Galactose.
   C. Starch.
   D. Proteins.
   E. Fats.

305. Of the following injuries or conditions, which will **not** be adequately protected by the use of moldable thermoplastic material?
   A. Femoral myositis ossificans

B. Iliotibial band friction syndrome

C. Fracture of the nasal bone

D. Sprain of the first carpometacarpal joint

E. Humeral exostosis

306. Osteoporosis is a condition that predominantly afflicts older women. Which of the following factors decreases the chance of developing this condition?

A. Moderate swimming and increased vitamin C intake

B. Weight-bearing activities and increased calcium intake

C. Maintaining 10 percent body fat and using a minimal-resistance stationary bike

D. Increased electrolytes and nonsteroidal anti-inflammatory medication

E. Avoidance of physical activity and dairy products

307. Deficiency symptoms may occur rapidly with diets suddenly low in

A. Vitamin A.

B. Iron.

C. Vitamin C.

D. Vitamin D.

E. Calcium.

308. The body's thermoregulatory system is controlled by the

A. Cerebral cortex.

B. Pons.

C. Cerebellum.

D. Hypothalmus.

E. Adrenal gland.

309. The common cold can play havoc with an entire team. Therefore, the prevention of colds is very important. Which of the following measures would help in preventing colds?

A. Taking antihistamines

B. Taking decongestants

C. Taking large doses of vitamin C

D. Avoiding extreme fatigue

E. Avoiding oversleeping

310. The form of flexibility exercise in which the muscle, or muscle group, is lengthened to its maximal length and held stationary is

A. Proprioceptive neuromuscular facilitation.

B. Dynamic stretching.

C. Plyometric stretching.

D. Static stretching.

E. Ballistic stretching.

311. Resistance activities in which the resistance is thrust is used to develop

A. Power.

B. Muscle definition.

C. Flexibility.

D. Accuracy.

E. Endurance.

312. The proper breathing pattern while performing a bench press is to

A. Inhale as the bar is thrust upward and exhale as the bar is lowered.

B. Hold the breath as the bar is lowered and inhale as the bar is thrust upward.

C. Inhale as the bar is lowered and exhale as the bar is thrust upward.

D. Hold the breath until one repetition is complete.

E. Inhale as the bar is lowered and hold the breath as the bar is thrust upward.

313. The vital capacity is a measure of the volume of air that

A. Is present in the lungs after the deepest possible inspiration.

B. Can be moved into and out of the lungs during the deepest possible breathing in excess of that breathed in and out normally.

C. Can be expelled by the most vigorous expiratory effort after the deepest possible inspiration.

D. Can be moved into and out of the lungs during normal respiration.

E. Remains in the lungs after the most vigorous expiratory effort.

314. Under which of the following combinations of environmental and physical conditions is an athlete most likely to be subject to hypothermia?

A. Air temperature of 30°F to 50°F, 50 percent humidity, and extreme fatigue

B. Air temperature of 30°F to 50°F, 80 percent humidity, and moderate fatigue

C. Air temperature of 20°F to 30°F, 50 percent humidity, and moderate fatigue

D. Air temperature of 30°F to 50°F, 80 percent humidity, and extreme fatigue

E. Air temperature of 20°F to 30°F, 30 percent humidity, and moderate fatigue

315. When a football helmet is fitted correctly, its posterior portion should
    A. Be at the level of the fourth cervical vertebrae when the neck is extended.
    B. Ride above the occipital bone.
    C. Be at the level of the sixth cervical vertebrae when the neck is extended.
    D. Cover the occipital bone.
    E. Be at the level of the fifth cervical vertebrae.

316. The biceps and anterior deltoid muscles perform what motion?
    A. Flexion
    B. Extension
    C. Abduction, glenohumeral
    D. Upward rotation
    E. Stabilization

317. When implementing conditioning programs for individuals 45 years or older, the first step should be
    A. Cooper's 12-minute walk-run test.
    B. The determination of the athlete's flexibility.
    C. A preparticipation medical screen.
    D. The determination of maximal oxygen consumption.
    E. Harvard step-test.

318. A basic principle involving the interrelationship of nutrients in the body is that
    A. Efficiency is directly proportional to the amount of nutrient present.
    B. A nutrient is involved in a singular reaction.
    C. No bodily reactions occur when excessive nutrients are ingested.
    D. Nutrients are required in specific ratios for optimum use.
    E. The body cannot use vegetable protein.

319. Which one of the following is responsible for retaining fluid in the tissues?
    A. Potassium ions
    B. Magnesium ions
    C. Calcium ions
    D. Hydrogen ions
    E. Sodium ions

320. The tendency for objects at rest to remain at rest and for objects in motion to remain in motion is covered by the law of
    A. Motion.
    B. Interaction.
    C. Inertia.
    D. Reaction.
    E. Physics.

321. Which one of the following would be the **most appropriate** program for preventing hamstring strains?
    A. Moist heat before workouts, group stretching exercises, and ice treatments after workouts
    B. Preseason endurance exercising, in-season interval training, and a postseason stretching program
    C. Preseason screening for muscular imbalances, midseason interval training, and late-season weight training and interval workouts
    D. Preseason screening for muscular imbalances, weight training programs to correct existing imbalances, and flexibility and stretching exercises
    E. Increasing electrolyte intake, in-season circuit training with emphasis on the lower extremity, and group stretching exercises.

The following scenario relates to questions 322 and 323: For the last 2 weeks one of your football players has been under the care of a physician for mononucleosis. The athlete is taking prednisone for his discomfort and consequently feels much better than at the onset of the symptoms. It is Wednesday of homecoming week, and the athlete comes to you, asking to be allowed to practice with the intention of playing in Saturday's game.

322. What is your response?
    A. Allow him to practice today
    B. Consult his parents before consenting to the player's participation
    C. Allow him to practice without pads in noncontact drills
    D. Palpate the abdomen to assess splenic enlargement
    E. Refer him to his physician

323. Once the attending physician has released the athlete to participate, how will you protect him from risk of internal injury?
    A. Require the athlete to wear a "flak jacket" while participating
    B. Have the athlete change to a position where there is less physical contact
    C. Restrict the athlete from participating in football
    D. Instruct the athlete in special techniques that limit his exposure to contact

E. Instruct the athlete to ice his upper left abdominal quadrant daily after practice

324. To prevent the transmission of bloodborne pathogens such as hepatitis B virus or human immunodeficiency virus, universal precautions must be taken with all of the following **except**
    A. Blood.
    B. Cerebrospinal fluid.
    C. Exudate.
    D. Blister fluid.
    E. Perspiration.

325. The contraction of the forearm extensors as the body is lowered in a push-up is an example of
    A. Isometric contraction.
    B. Isotonic contraction.
    C. Concentric contraction.
    D. Eccentric contraction.
    E. Motor contraction.

326. Statistically, as body weight increases, there is a significant increase in
    A. Premature deaths.
    B. Life expectancy.
    C. Mental retardation.
    D. Accidents.
    E. Drownings.

327. Which of the following is not a reason for flexibility conditioning?
    A. Stress
    B. Injury prevention
    C. Skill
    D. Agility
    E. Range of motion

328. After a knee injury and before competition, an athlete should condition the injured area to have proper
    A. Strength, range of motion, and flexibility.
    B. Strength, flexibility, and laxity.
    C. Range of motion, girth, and laxity.
    D. Girth, flexibility, and agility.
    E. Range of motion, flexibility, and endurance.

329. Which of the following factors does not affect the speed with which alcohol enters the blood?
    A. The amount of food in the stomach
    B. The time of day
    C. How quickly the alcohol is consumed

D. The chemical make-up of the body
E. The type of alcohol consumed

330. Of the following activities, the one especially good for cardiovascular fitness is
    A. Softball.
    B. Weight training.
    C. Golf.
    D. Jumping rope.
    E. High jumping.

331. Which of the following are described as biconcave disks?
    A. Red blood cells
    B. Leukocytes
    C. Platelets
    D. Alveoli
    E. Lymphocytes

332. The area of dead heart muscle that results from a blocked artery is called
    A. Myocardial infarction.
    B. Angina pectoris.
    C. Embolus.
    D. Coronary thrombosis.
    E. Atherosclerosis.

333. Fatty deposits that restrict the flow of blood through arteries are characteristics of
    A. Arteriosclerosis.
    B. Phlebitis.
    C. Atherosclerosis.
    D. Coronary thrombosis.
    E. Embolus.

334. The expulsion of semisolid wastes from the large intestine relates to which function?
    A. Digestion
    B. Secretion
    C. Motility
    D. Absorption
    E. Elimination

335. The team physician tells an athlete that a lump under the arm is a benign tumor. This means that the athlete
    A. Has a localized form of cancer.
    B. Has lymphoma.
    C. Does not have cancer.
    D. Should undergo radiation therapy.
    E. Should undergo chemotherapy.

336. The amount of energy used by the body at rest is called
    A. Calories.
    B. Normal temperature.
    C. Caloric balance.
    D. Basal metabolic rate.
    E. Metabolic equivalents.

337. One of the most popular amphetamines is
    A. Cocaine.
    B. Heroin.
    C. Marijuana.
    D. Ecstasy.
    E. Methadone.

338. Which of the following is most commonly used by people who want to stay awake for long periods of time?
    A. Hallucinogens
    B. Antibiotics
    C. Sedatives
    D. Amphetamines
    E. Analgesics

339. A symptom not found in deficiencies of B vitamins is
    A. Diarrhea.
    B. Dementia.
    C. Dental caries.
    D. Dermatitis.
    E. Death.

340. Which of the following would the physician prescribe to help sleep?
    A. Hallucinogens
    B. Antibiotics
    C. Barbiturates
    D. Amphetamines
    E. Analgesics

341. Excess fat puts extra strain on the circulatory system because
    A. It causes diabetes.
    B. It requires the digestive system to work harder.
    C. It causes a lack of exercise.
    D. It requires body muscles to work harder.
    E. It is a poor form of energy.

342. To determine the degree of fatness, an athletic trainer may
    A. Measure skin folds with calipers.
    B. Pinch the calf of the patient's leg.
    C. Take the patient's blood pressure.
    D. Determine how much the patient eats.
    E. Determine the patient's metabolic rate.

343. The ability to maintain physical effort over a period of time is called
    A. Overload.
    B. Flexibility.
    C. Endurance.
    D. Tonus.
    E. Clonus.

344. A program of regular exercise
    A. Is not necessary if you eat a balanced diet.
    B. Increases your capacity for activity.
    C. Is important only for people over 40.
    D. Is less important today than it was 50 years ago.
    E. Reduces your metabolic rate.

345. Ten minutes after your workout, your pulse is 105. Which of the following statements is true?
    A. You are in good shape.
    B. You are probably a woman.
    C. You have overexerted yourself.
    D. You probably have diabetes.
    E. You are having a myocardial infarction.

346. You are skiing down a remote slope when you come across someone who has broken a leg and is partially buried in the snow. The skier has been there for more than an hour and is close to coma because so much body heat has been lost. You should not give the skier an alcoholic drink as a "warm up" because
    A. The skier might become intoxicated.
    B. Alcohol causes a loss of body heat.
    C. Alcohol cannot be metabolized by the body.
    D. Alcohol has no nutrients.
    E. Alcohol might warm the skier up too much.

347. Movement of the foot before striking the football during a punt relates to which motion?
    A. Supination
    B. Dorsiflexion
    C. Plantar flexion
    D. Eversion
    E. Extension

348. The greatest overall cause of stress is
    A. Death or serious illness.
    B. Financial ruin.
    C. Anxiety or depression.
    D. Change.
    E. Marriage.

349. Today, health is measured in terms of
    A. Total absence of disease.
    B. Lack of mental problems.
    C. The quality of effective and enjoyable living.
    D. Physical fitness.
    E. Orthopedic stability.

350. What bone is included as part of the roof of the orbit?
    A. Sphenoid
    B. Ethmoid
    C. Zygomatic
    D. Lacrimal
    E. Palatine

351. A person who wants to lose at least 1 pound a week should reduce his or her daily caloric intake by how many calories?
    A. 100
    B. 200
    C. 500
    D. 1000
    E. 2000

352. Through which of the following factors would left-sided heart failure affect gas exchange at the pulmonary membrane?
    A. Gas pressure differences
    B. Cross-sectional area
    C. Membrane thickness
    D. Diffusion coefficient of gases
    E. Disease state

353. Compared with nonsmokers, cigarette smokers tend to have
    A. The same mortality rate.
    B. Lower morbidity rate of cancer.
    C. A greater life expectancy.
    D. A shorter life expectancy.
    E. Better general health.

354. The early signs of skin cancer include
    A. Changes in moles or skin blemishes.
    B. Mild intestinal upset.
    C. Chronic fatigue.
    D. Hot flashes.
    E. Chest pain.

355. What is a sufficient amount of milk for most adults?
    A. 4 cups a day
    B. 3 cups a day
    C. 2 cups a day
    D. 1 cup a day
    E. 0 cups a day

356. How many servings of foods from the fruit and vegetable group do adults need each day?
    A. 0
    B. 1
    C. 2
    D. 3
    E. 4

357. When a person is in very good physical condition, his or her heart
    A. Pumps faster.
    B. Pumps less blood at once.
    C. Pumps more slowly.
    D. Pumps with increased irregularity.
    E. Pumps more sporadically.

358. A stroke occurs when blood cannot get to the
    A. Myocardium.
    B. Kidneys.
    C. Brain.
    D. Superior vena cava.
    E. Lungs.

359. It takes approximately how many calories to make a pound of fat?
    A. 1000
    B. 1800
    C. 2500
    D. 3500
    E. 7000

360. A condition resulting from the ingestion of too many vitamins is called
    A. Euhydration.
    B. Malnutrition.
    C. Kwashiorkor.
    D. Hypervitaminosis.
    E. Hypovitaminosis.

361. The drug curare exerts its action in the
    A. Receptor region.
    B. Conductile region.
    C. Transmissional region.
    D. Contractile region.
    E. Motor region.

362. Most common nutritional deficiencies of the American diet can be corrected by including more of which food groups?
    A. Proteins and amino acids
    B. Carbohydrates
    C. Fruits and vegetables
    D. Milk and milk products
    E. Salts and sugars

363. The best sources of vitamin C are
    A. Beef, poultry, and fish.
    B. Breads, cereal, and cookies.
    C. Citrus fruits, potatoes, and tomatoes.
    D. Liver, heart, and kidney meats.
    E. Milk, cheese, and yogurt.

364. The four basic food groups are
    A. Meat, fish, milk, and bread and cereal.
    B. Meat, milk, fruit and vegetables, and bread and cereal.
    C. Meat, fruit and vegetables, bread and cereal, and fish.
    D. Meat, vegetables, fruit, and cereal.
    E. Meat, poultry, fruit, and vegetables.

365. Babies born to mothers who smoke
    A. Have an increased incidence of psychological problems.
    B. Have a shorter life span.
    C. Tend to weigh less.
    D. Eventually become addicted to cigarettes.
    E. Are born with emphysema.

366. The average athlete in training has a daily caloric need of
    A. 1500–2000 cal.
    B. 2500–3000 cal.
    C. 4500–5000 cal.
    D. 5500–6000 cal.
    E. 6500–7200 cal.

367. What percentage of calories should come from carbohydrates in a normal, well-balanced diet?
    A. 5%–10%
    B. 15%–20%
    C. 25%–30%
    D. 50%–60%
    E. 75%–80%

368. Which of the following is a false statement regarding vitamins?
    A. Vitamins can be harmful.
    B. Supplements do not make up for skipped breakfast.
    C. Brand names are better than less expensive ones.
    D. There is no difference between natural and synthetic vitamins.
    E. A condition resulting from ingesting too many vitamins is called hypervitaminosis.

369. Vomiting relates to which function?
    A. Digestion
    B. Secretion
    C. Motility
    D. Absorption
    E. Elimination

370. Which of the following is false regarding carbohydrates?
    A. Mainly used for energy
    B. May be synthesized into amino acids and some fatty acids
    C. Require less energy to oxidize than do other energy nutrients
    D. Have the greatest caloric content per gram of the energy nutrients
    E. Do not have the greatest caloric content per gram of the energy nutrients

371. The chief source of inexpensive energy, fiber, B vitamins, and iron is
    A. Meat.
    B. Fruits and vegetables.
    C. Milk.
    D. Breads and cereals.
    E. Fish and poultry.

372. Which vitamin is found only in animal sources and should be supplemented in vegetarian diets?
    A. B_1
    B. B_2
    C. Niacin
    D. B_6
    E. B_{12}

373. The Recommended Daily Allowance (RDA) for iron is relatively high because
    A. With many nutrients, an intake for iron above the RDA is excreted rather than being stored.
    B. Rather large amounts of iron are excreted or lost, especially by menstruating women.
    C. The body requires large iron intakes to replace red blood cells.
    D. The human body is rather inefficient in using iron in foods.
    E. The body absorbs comparatively little of the iron in foods.

374. Cortisone is a/an
    A. Pain killer.
    B. Anti-inflammatory agent.
    C. Anticoagulant.
    D. Enzyme.
    E. Analgesic.

375. The level of glucose circulating in the bloodstream depends primarily on the proper functioning of
    A. Bile secreted from the gallbladder.
    B. Amylase action on starch.
    C. The liver and insulin levels.
    D. The adrenal glands.
    E. The kidneys.

376. The postovulatory temperature rise occurs during
    A. Ovulation.
    B. The follicular phase.
    C. The luteal phase.
    D. The menstrual flow.
    E. The premenstrual phase.

377. Swallowing relates to which function?
    A. Digestion
    B. Secretion
    C. Motility
    D. Absorption
    E. Elimination

378. Weight gain results from
    A. Consuming a diet in which a high percentage of calories is from carbohydrates.
    B. Consuming a diet in which a high percentage of calories is from fat.
    C. Consuming a diet in which a high percentage of calories is from protein.
    D. Positive energy balance.
    E. Negative energy balance.

379. Digestion of starch begins in the
    A. Esophagus.
    B. Mouth.
    C. Stomach.
    D. Large intestine.
    E. Small intestine.

380. The chief source of the nutrient riboflavin and of vitamin D is which of the following groups?
    A. Meat
    B. Fruit and vegetables
    C. Milk
    D. Bread and cereal
    E. Fat and oil

381. The corpus luteum remains active during the first trimester of pregnancy because of the action of
    A. A pituitary gonadotropin.
    B. A chorionic gonadotropin.
    C. Estrogen.
    D. Prolactin.
    E. Progesterone.

382. Most ascorbic acid comes from which group?
    A. Meat
    B. Fruit and vegetables
    C. Milk
    D. Bread and cereal
    E. Fat and oil

383. A neuron, motor end plate, and included muscle fibers are the parts of
    A. An egocentric philonome.
    B. A motor unit.
    C. A synapse.
    D. A ginglymoid articulation.
    E. A myotome.

384. An excess of glucose in the blood causes the secretion of
    A. Thyroxine.
    B. Insulin.
    C. Glycogen.
    D. Adrenalin.
    E. Thiamine.

385. Oxygen concentration of the blood relates to a/an
  A. Chemoreceptor.
  B. Electromagnetic receptor.
  C. Thermoreceptor.
  D. Mechanoreceptor.
  E. Sensitoreceptor.

386. The carbohydrate not digested or absorbed by humans is
  A. Insulin.
  B. Glycogen.
  C. Cellulose.
  D. Starch.
  E. Glucose.

387. The triceps and posterior deltoids perform what motion?
  A. Flexion
  B. Extension
  C. Abduction, glenohumeral
  D. Adduction, glenohumeral
  E. Stabilization

388. The contraction of the forearm flexors as the body is lowered during a pull-up is an example of
  A. Isometric contraction.
  B. Isotonic contraction.
  C. Concentric contraction.
  D. Eccentric contraction.
  E. Motor contraction.

389. French fries may have more vitamin C than potato chips have because
  A. They are cooked at a lower temperature.
  B. They are more stable to alkali.
  C. The potatoes are cooked in their skins.
  D. Less of their surface is exposed to oxygen and light.
  E. Ascorbic acid is water soluable.

390. Hydrochloric acid in the stomach is
  A. An emulsifying agent.
  B. A digestive enzyme.
  C. A promoter of mineral use.
  D. Secreted in greater amounts in pernicious anemia.
  E. A neutralizer.

391. Clotting of blood does not depend on
  A. Calcium.
  B. Vitamin K.
  C. Thrombin.
  D. Fibrinogen.
  E. Vitamin E.

392. One ounce of protein has the same number of calories as
  A. 1 ounce of meat.
  B. 1 ounce of fat.
  C. 1 ounce of sugar.
  D. 1 ounce of cholesterol.
  E. 1 ounce of milk.

393. Significant digestion of fat begins in the
  A. Esophagus.
  B. Mouth.
  C. Stomach.
  D. Large intestine.
  E. Small intestine.

394. Maximum oxygen uptake for world-class distance runners is approximately
  A. 30 mL/kg/min.
  B. 40 mL/kg/min.
  C. 60 mL/kg/min.
  D. 80 mL/kg/min.
  E. 100 mL/kg/min.

395. A nonessential amino acid
  A. Is not used in protein synthesis in the human body.
  B. Is used for protein synthesis but can be formed from other substances.
  C. Must be supplied by food.
  D. Has no function in the human body.
  E. Is supplied only by the human body.

396. If angular velocity were constant, a longer lever would expand the range of motion, but
  A. It would require more force.
  B. It would require more mass.
  C. No difference would exist.
  D. It would require greater acceleration.
  E. It would require less acceleration.

397. While hiking you find it necessary to jump from a 3-foot-high boulder to the ground below. For best balance you should land
  A. In a deep squat position with your weight forward.
  B. In a bent-knee position with weight directly over the feet.

C. With your weight back so that the hands may be used for support if necessary.

D. With your torso forward to absorb the shock to the knees.

E. With your hands forward.

398. Iron, phosphorus, and B vitamins are produced in significant amounts by the _____ group.
  A. Meat
  B. Fruit and vegetable
  C. Milk
  D. Bread and cereal
  E. Fat and oil

399. Which nutrients will need to be added first to the diet of a breastfed baby?
  A. None is critical
  B. Vitamin C and protein
  C. Calcium and phosphorus
  D. Thiamine and riboflavin
  E. Vitamin C and iron

400. Splitting of glucose into two 3-carbon molecules involves
  A. Glycolysis.
  B. The Krebs cycle.
  C. An electron transport chain.
  D. Glycogen formation.
  E. Enzymatic release.

401. What is the caloric content of 100 g of ground beef that is about 45% water, 23% protein, and 32% fat?
  A. 130 kcal
  B. 380 kcal
  C. 220 kcal
  D. 530 kcal
  E. 620 kcal

402. Which of the following is a mineral that plays a role in carbohydrate metabolism?
  A. Iron
  B. Insulin
  C. Zinc
  D. Thyroxine
  E. Calcium

403. Proliferation of the uterine lining during the female menstrual cycle appears to depend most directly on
  A. Follicle-stimulating hormone
  B. Luteotropic hormone.
  C. Progesterone.

D. Estrogen.

E. Human chorionic gonadotropin.

404. The contraction of the forearm flexors as the body is pulled up during a pull-up is an example of
  A. Isometric contraction.
  B. Isotonic contraction.
  C. Concentric contraction.
  D. Eccentric contraction.
  E. Motor contraction.

405. Labels on some foods indicate that they contain hydrogenated fat. This refers to a process that makes the fats
  A. Slightly lower in kilocalories.
  B. More nutritious.
  C. More saturated.
  D. Liquid at room temperature.
  E. More unsaturated.

406. The nutrient that cannot be made in the body is
  A. Cholesterol.
  B. Vitamin D.
  C. Vitamin K.
  D. Glycogen.
  E. Linoleic acid.

407. Most of the carbon dioxide generated in cellular metabolism is transported in the blood in the form of
  A. Carbaminohemoglobin.
  B. Bicarbonate.
  C. Carbonic acid.
  D. Dissolved carbon dioxide.
  E. Reabsorbed acid.

408. In order for amino acids to be built into proteins, they must be
  A. Transaminated.
  B. Deaminated.
  C. Oxidized.
  D. Essential.
  E. In excess of energy needs.

409. Bile is
  A. An emulsifier of proteins.
  B. Important for the absorption of fat-soluble vitamins.
  C. A fat-splitting enzyme.
  D. Important for the transport of glucose.
  E. Important for the secretion of insulin.

410. Of the following factors, water balance is primarily controlled by
    A. Fluid intake.
    B. Perspiration.
    C. The concentration of minerals.
    D. The amount of urine.
    E. The acid-base balance.

411. The level of glucose circulating in the bloodstream depends primarily on the proper functioning of
    A. Bile secreted from the gallbladder.
    B. Amylase action on starch.
    C. The liver and insulin levels.
    D. The adrenal glands.
    E. Intestinal hydrolysis.

412. The Cori cycle allows skeletal muscle lactic acid to be
    A. Oxidized to carbon dioxide and water by skeletal muscles.
    B. Oxidized to carbon dioxide and water by the liver.
    C. Used in generating glucose at the liver.
    D. Used in generating pyruvic acid by the heart.
    E. Broken down into a usable form of pyruvic acid.

413. The three monosaccharides important in nutrition are
    A. Glucose, sucrose, and fructose.
    B. Galactose fructose, and lactose.
    C. Maltose, lactose, and sucrose.
    D. Glucose, fructose, and galactose.
    E. Glucose, galactose, and sucrose.

414. Immunity to disease depends most on the body's
    A. Carbohydrates.
    B. Lipids.
    C. Proteins.
    D. Vitamins.
    E. Fats.

415. All but one of the following measures is often effective in lowering blood cholesterol level.
    A. Lower cholesterol intake
    B. Lower total fat intake
    C. Lower polyunsaturated fat intake
    D. Lower saturated fat intake
    E. Lower total calorie intake

416. Colostrum is different from true milk because it contains
    A. Extra enzymes.
    B. Higher levels of protein.
    C. More lactose or milk sugar.
    D. More lipids.
    E. More carbohydrates.

417. When nutrients enter the blood vessels from the small intestine, they are first transported to
    A. The liver.
    B. The kidney.
    C. All cells of the body.
    D. The thoracic duct.
    E. The pancreas.

418. The term *distal* refers to which of the following?
    A. Toward the feet
    B. Away from the midline of the body
    C. Away from the trunk
    D. Front portion of the body
    E. Toward the midline of the body

419. If a person lacks the enzyme lactase, what will be the consequence?
    A. He or she will be unable to digest table sugar.
    B. His or her maltase and sucrase will compensate for the lack of lactase.
    C. He or she will be unable to absorb glucose.
    D. He or she will be unable to digest milk.
    E. He or she will be unable to digest proteins.

420. When the three energy nutrients are completely oxidized, the product(s) common to all three areas is/are
    A. Pyrovic acid.
    B. Urea.
    C. Carbon dioxide, water, adenosine triphosphate.
    D. Adenosine triphosphate.
    E. Carbon dioxide, water, adenosine triphosphate, and urea.

421. The inborn biological mechanism that governs energy intake automatically is
    A. Appetite.
    B. Hunger.
    C. Calorimetry.
    D. Survival.
    E. Hyperphagia.

422. The anterior serratus muscle performs what motion?
    A. Adduction, scapular
    B. Abduction, scapular
    C. Internal rotation
    D. External rotation
    E. Stabilization

423. Thiamine is associated with
    A. Formation of red blood cells.
    B. Blood coagulation.
    C. Collagen formation.
    D. Energy release from energy nutrients.
    E. Formation of mucopolysaccharides.

424. The cooking principles applied to the preservation of thiamine may also be applied to the preservation of
    A. Vitamin A.
    B. Ascorbic acid.
    C. Valine.
    D. Vitamin K.
    E. Vitamin E.

425. Milk provides about one half of this nutrient available to the U.S. population.
    A. Thiamine
    B. Folic acid
    C. Riboflavin
    D. Biotin
    E. Pantothenic acid

426. Vitamin A is needed for
    A. Converting vitamin D to a usable form.
    B. Synthesis of some hormones.
    C. Maintaining the integrity of mucous membranes.
    D. Blood clotting.
    E. Immunity.

427. Vitamin B deficiencies cause lack of energy because
    A. A lack of oxygen, which is needed for energy metabolism, results.
    B. A lack of coenzymes, which are needed for energy metabolism, results.
    C. The B vitamins are an energy source for humans.
    D. They affect the brain and therefore make people feel tired.

    E. They decrease the distribution of glucose to the cells, thereby causing fatigue.

428. Which of the following body processes does not depend directly on the presence of calcium in the body fluids?
    A. Blood clotting
    B. Muscle relaxation
    C. Transmission of nerve impulses
    D. Deposition of calcium in the bones
    E. Transport of oxygen

429. A symptom of a deficiency of which of the following nutrients would take the longest to develop?
    A. Thiamine
    B. Riboflavin
    C. Ascorbic acid
    D. Vitamin A
    E. Niacin

430. What is the name of cranial nerve IV?
    A. Abducent
    B. Optic
    C. Trochlear
    D. Olfactory
    E. Oculomotor

431. The absolute refractory period is in the
    A. Receptor region.
    B. Conductile region.
    C. Transmissional region.
    D. Contractile region.
    E. Motor region.

432. In the adult, deficiency of vitamin D causes a condition known as
    A. Xerophthalmia.
    B. Rickets.
    C. Osteomalacia.
    D. Beriberi.
    E. Osteoporosis.

433. Which nutrient increases the absorption of calcium from the intestinal tract?
    A. Biotin
    B. Vitamin B_{12}
    C. Vitamin A
    D. Iron
    E. Vitamin D

434. Which of the following is the poorest source of iron?
  A. Meat
  B. Raisins
  C. Milk
  D. Enriched cereals
  E. Nuts

435. Bulk in the diet is derived from which food source?
  A. Lipids
  B. Proteins
  C. Lipoproteins
  D. Carbohydrates
  E. Fats, oils

436. To nourish the body is to nourish
  A. The brain.
  B. The liver.
  C. Individual cells.
  D. The stomach.
  E. The appetite.

437. Which of the following would not come under the category of empty calorie foods?
  A. Peanuts
  B. Potato chips
  C. Candy
  D. Cola drinks
  E. Coffee with sugar

438. During the life cycle, the need for protein is greatest
  A. When one is engaged in athletics.
  B. During rapid growth, as in childhood.
  C. In old age.
  D. During adulthood.
  E. In infancy.

439. Subject A has a respiratory rate of 14 respirations per minute and a tidal volume of 475 mL per breath. Subject A's minute respiratory volume would be
  A. 4750 mL/min.
  B. 6550 mL/min.
  C. 6650 mL/min.
  D. 7650 mL/min.
  E. 6750 mL/min.

440. Cobalt is a component of
  A. Thiamine.
  B. Riboflavin.
  C. Vitamin B_6.
  D. Vitamin B_{12}.
  E. Niacin.

441. When lipid consumption is in excess of body needs, the excess lipid is
  A. Stored as fat only.
  B. Stored as glycogen only.
  C. Stored as glycogen and fat.
  D. Not absorbed from the small intestine.
  E. Excreted in the urine.

442. Adequate nutrition is most likely ensured by
  A. The use of vitamin supplements.
  B. Spending more money on food.
  C. The selection of high nutrient-dense food.
  D. Waterless methods of cookery.
  E. A diet comprising the basic four food groups.

443. The trapezius and rhomboid muscles perform what motion?
  A. Adduction, scapular
  B. Abduction, scapular
  C. Internal rotation
  D. External rotation
  E. Stabilization

444. Which factor usually accounts for wide variations in energy expenditure of adults of similar age, size, and sex?
  A. Type of diet consumed.
  B. Physical activity.
  C. Climate.
  D. Mental work.
  E. Basal metabolism.

445. The part of a plant that may contribute substantial amounts of calcium and iron is/are the
  A. Root.
  B. Stem.
  C. Green leaves.
  D. Blossoms.
  E. Seeds.

446. Foods must be carefully selected for vitamin C content. Therefore, which of the following, in standard amounts, contributes about the same amount of ascorbic acid as a serving of orange juice?
  A. Celery or tomatoes
  B. Carrots or potatoes

C. Apple juice or apricot nectar

D. Pear or peach

E. Broccoli or cantaloupe

447. Chylomicrons

A. Are resynthesized fat molecules that are absorbed into the lymph.

B. Are small droplets of fat that remain in the digestive tube until they are removed with the feces.

C. Are similar to the water-insoluble micelles.

D. Are the same as bile salts.

E. Are a product of fat breakdown derived from salt and water.

448. In the United States today, the most common nutrition problem of adults is

A. Iron-deficiency anemia.

B. Vitamin A deficiency.

C. Insufficient physical activity.

D. Atherosclerosis.

E. Obesity.

449. Movement of the lower arm during a pull-up involves which of the following motions?

A. Flexion

B. Extension

C. Supination

D. Pronation

E. Rotation

450. Calculate the energy value of this meal:

FOOD	PROTEIN	FAT	CHO
One hamburger	17 g	22 g	40 g
One large cola			25 g
One order French fries	4 g	14 g	40 g

The number of calories from carbohydrates was

A. 105.

B. 189.

C. 420.

D. 750.

E. 945.

451. It takes _____ for a person to get in optimum aerobic condition.

A. 18–21 days

B. 34 weeks

C. 68 weeks

D. 3 months

E. 2 weeks

452. Most authorities in sports medicine consider one of the most important objectives in conditioning athletes to be

A. Warm-up.

B. Flexibility.

C. Cooldown.

D. Routine.

E. Determination.

453. One objective in blister care is to reduce friction. Which of the following supplies does not reduce friction?

A. Moleskin

B. Skin lube

C. 1½-inch white tape

D. Dermiclear

E. Combine roll

454. Which of the following is not a reason for strength conditioning?

A. Prevention of injuries

B. Protection of injured area

C. Development of definition

D. Development of skills

E. Development of strength

455. Which of the following best describes the goal of "gradualism"?

A. To develop conditioning levels by certain deadlines

B. To spread out injury rehabilitation to prevent aggravating the injury.

C. To progress gradually from warm-up to flexibility to strength conditioning.

D. To ensure that no workout will severely overstress the athlete.

E. To gradually cool down after strength conditioning.

456. Which of the following is not related to warm-up activities?

A. To develop permanent and progressively increasing functional ranges of motion

B. To increase heart rate

C. To increase body temperature

D. To increase cardiac circulation

E. To increase respiratory rate

457. Resistance activities should improve strength in areas needed to improve skill and
    A. Prevent injuries.
    B. Give muscle definition.
    C. Increase body weight.
    D. Develop symmetry.
    E. Accuracy.

458. Activities in preseason that put a lot of stress on body parts should start very easy and progress
    A. Slowly to slightly less than the sport demands.
    B. Quickly to slightly less than the sport demands.
    C. Slowly to as much or more than the sport demands.
    D. Quickly to as much or more than the sport demands.
    E. Quickly to exceed what the sport demands.

459. An athlete may increase or develop physical work capacity most efficiently by
    A. Running and lifting daily.
    B. Running and lifting on alternate days.
    C. Dieting and lifting.
    D. Using overload principles progressively.
    E. Dieting and running on alternate days.

460. What soft tissue structure lies under McBurney's point?
    A. Liver
    B. Spleen
    C. Bladder
    D. Gallbladder
    E. Appendix

461. An effective weight-reduction program must
    A. Change basic eating and exercise patterns.
    B. Reduce weight at more than 10 pounds a month.
    C. Reduce weight at more than 25 pounds a month.
    D. Provide calories in excess of the dieter's energy requirements.
    E. Include a protein-only diet.

462. Trauma means
    A. Tissue reaction to injury.
    B. Rapid onset.
    C. Fatigue.
    D. An injury or wound.
    E. An injury with rapid onset of swelling.

463. What does tensile strength mean, for example, when referring to the quality of athletic tape?
    A. How difficult it is to tear
    B. The number of cloth fibers per square inch
    C. The elastic quality of the 6-inch elastic wrap
    D. How well it sticks to the skin
    E. How long it sticks to the skin

464. For cardiovascular fitness to occur, the exercise needs to last at least 20 minutes while maintaining the
    A. Maximum pulse rate.
    B. Minimum pulse rate.
    C. Target pulse rate.
    D. Maximum respiratory rate.
    E. Maximum lactate rate.

465. What bones form the ankle joint?
    A. Talus, navicular, calcaneous
    B. Tibia, fibula, talus
    C. Tibia, navicular, fibula
    D. Tibia, fibula, calcaneous
    E. Talus, calcaneous, fibula

466. Adipose tissue is
    A. Connective tissue that secretes lubrication.
    B. Connective tissue that attaches to bones and ligaments.
    C. Epithelial tissue that insulates and stores energy.
    D. Connective tissue that serves as insulation and stores energy.
    E. Nervous tissue that transmits afferent impulses.

467. Name the two structures that pass through Guyon's canal.
    A. Ulnar nerve and artery
    B. Radial nerve and artery
    C. Radial nerve and ulnar nerve
    D. Radial artery and ulnar artery
    E. Radial nerve and ulnar artery

468. The muscle that everts the foot is the
    A. Peroneal
    B. Long extensor of the great toe
    C. Anterior tibial
    D. Posterior tibial
    E. Long flexor of the great toe

469. What is the cause of hard corns?
    A. Friction
    B. Pressure
    C. Extra callus
    D. Virus
    E. Force of walking

470. What structure is most likely to be injured when a varus stress is put on the knee?
    A. Medial collateral ligament
    B. Medial meniscus
    C. Lateral collateral ligament
    D. Lateral meniscus
    E. Anterior cruciate ligament

471. The rotator cuff is a
    A. Ligament.
    B. Joint.
    C. Group of muscles.
    D. Tendon.
    E. Bone.

472. Poor throwing technique (not following through all the way) can cause strain or irritation to what structure?
    A. Biceps tendon
    B. Deltoid muscle
    C. Triceps muscle
    D. Acromioclavicular ligament
    E. Biceps muscle

473. The weakest aspect of the ankle is
    A. That it is a hinge joint.
    B. Its ligamentous support.
    C. Its thin articular capsule.
    D. Its muscular arrangement.
    E. Its small size in comparison to other joints.

474. Good foot care includes
    A. Wearing high tops.
    B. Wearing shoes that are the proper size and socks.
    C. Powdering the feet twice a day.
    D. Wearing arch supports.
    E. Application of skin lube.

475. Which of the following is used as a base for stirrups?
    A. Tie in
    B. Heel locks
    C. Anchor strips

476. The dorsal cavity consists of
    A. Cranial and abdominal cavities.
    B. Cranial and thoracic cavities.
    C. Spinal and abdominal cavities.
    D. Cranial and spinal cavities.
    E. Thoracic and abdominal cavities.

477. The epiphyseal line injuries are dangerous in early adolescence because they disrupt
    A. Tendon integrity.
    B. Growth centers.
    C. Circulation.
    D. Lymphatic distribution.
    E. Pimples.

478. The anterior cruciate ligament stabilizes the knee joint to prevent the
    A. Femur from moving anteriorly on the tibia.
    B. Tibia from moving anteriorly on the femur.
    C. Tibia from moving posteriorly on the femur.
    D. Femur from moving posteriorly on the tibia.
    E. Patella from moving anteriorly over the tibia.

479. Jumping jack (movement of the arms) is done in which plane?
    A. Frontal
    B. Transverse
    C. Sagittal
    D. Medial
    E. Lateral

480. All of these structures run through the cubital fossa except the
    A. Biceps tendon.
    B. Median nerve.
    C. Ulnar nerve.
    D. Brachial artery.
    E. Musculocutaneous nerve.

481. When the knee is hyperextended, the ligament most susceptible to injury is the
    A. Patellar.
    B. Anterior cruciate.
    C. Lateral collateral.
    D. Medial collateral.
    E. Posterior cruciate.

482. Knee braces
    A. Have demonstrated excellent ability to enhance joint stability.
    B. Have demonstrated no ability to enhance joint stability.
    C. Can protect the joint from cartilage damage but not from collateral ligament damage.
    D. Can protect the joint from collateral ligament damage but not from cartilage damage.
    E. Have demonstrated little effectiveness in athletics.

483. Deficiency of several nutrients can result in anemia or can make anemia more likely. A deficiency of which of the following nutrients is **least** likely to be associated with anemia?
    A. Thiamine
    B. Folic acid
    C. Vitamin B_{12}
    D. Vitamin C
    E. Cobalt

484. The entity most responsible for arm problems in throwing activities is
    A. Improper technique.
    B. Too long a warm-up.
    C. Gradualism in training.
    D. Lack of strength.
    E. Lack of endurance.

485. Which of the following compounds cannot be formed from fatty acids?
    A. Triglycerides
    B. Carbon dioxide
    C. Acetylcoenzyme A
    D. Glucose
    E. Ketones

486. Which condition would present the greatest risk to an athlete participating in a collision sport?
    A. Spondylo
    B. Spondylosis
    C. Spondylolysis
    D. Spondylolysthesis
    E. Scoliosis

487. Which part of the tooth is very sensitive?
    A. Dentin
    B. Enamel
    C. Pulp
    D. Gum
    E. Root

488. During stress exercise, many physiological changes occur. Among these changes is
    A. Skeletal atrophy.
    B. Osteoporosis.
    C. Skeletal hypertrophy.
    D. Osteochondritis.
    E. Increased bone density.

489. When taping most areas, the athletic trainer should start with
    A. Anchors.
    B. Heel locks.
    C. Figure eights.
    D. Lock strips.
    E. Horseshoes.

490. The effectiveness of tape in supporting a joint is
    A. Unknown.
    B. Best after 15 minutes of warm-up.
    C. Better in younger athletes.
    D. Indispensable in preventing injuries.
    E. Only because of limiting range of motion.

491. Pull-up (movement of the arms) is done in which plane?
    A. Sagittal
    B. Frontal
    C. Transverse
    D. Medial
    E. Lateral

492. Which of the following statements is false regarding selection of tape size and type?
    A. Narrower tape is used for smaller body parts.
    B. Elastic tapes are chosen to encircle muscle mass or for better conformity.
    C. Nonelastic tapes encircling a muscle belly will reduce circulation.
    D. Narrower tape is used for larger body parts.
    E. Leukotape is more adhesive, is more rigid, has greater tensile strength, and is more expensive than is cloth tape.

493. The forehand drive in tennis (movement of the criterion arm) is performed in which plane?
    A. Frontal
    B. Sagittal
    C. Transverse
    D. Medial
    E. Lateral

494. In the initial phase of throwing a ball, as the shoulder girdle and arm move from a posterior retracted position to a forward, internally rotated position, the primary muscles responsible for moving the scapulae and the arm forward are the

    A. Subscapular, anterior deltoid, coracobrachial, and anterior serratus

    B. Supraspinous, teres major, rhomboids, and greater pectoral

    C. Anterior serratus, subscapular, anterior deltoid, and greater pectoral

    D. Anterior serratus, upper trapezius, latissimus dorsi, and greater pectoral

    E. Subscapular, upper trapezius, latissimus dorsi, and triceps

ANSWERS FOR SAMPLE WRITTEN QUESTIONS

DOMAIN I: PREVENTION

1. A	35. D	69. A	103. D	137. B
2. B	36. C	70. D	104. C	138. C
3. A	37. A	71. B	105. E	139. B
4. A	38. B	72. D	106. A	140. D
5. D	39. B	73. A	107. B	141. B
6. A	40. C	74. C	108. E	142. C
7. B	41. A	75. D	109. B	143. A
8. D	42. A	76. B	110. B	144. B
9. B	43. B	77. B	111. A	145. C
10. A	44. B	78. C	112. B	146. A
11. E	45. C	79. B	113. B	147. B
12. C	46. C	80. C	114. C	148. A
13. C	47. D	81. C	115. B	149. B
14. A	48. B	82. A	116. A	150. A
15. B	49. C	83. B	117. B	151. D
16. B	50. E	84. C	118. C	152. A
17. B	51. B	85. C	119. C	153. B
18. C	52. B	86. C	120. C	154. C
19. C	53. B	87. B	121. A	155. B
20. A	54. D	88. B	122. A	156. D
21. A	55. B	89. C	123. B	157. C
22. A	56. C	90. C	124. A	158. C
23. C	57. B	91. B	125. D	159. A
24. E	58. A	92. A	126. B	160. C
25. D	59. B	93. B	127. D	161. D
26. C	60. B	94. D	128. A	162. B
27. B	61. E	95. A	129. D	163. D
28. A	62. E	96. D	130. D	164. D
29. A	63. C	97. A	131. B	165. C
30. D	64. C	98. B	132. A	166. A
31. D	65. A	99. B	133. C	167. C
32. C	66. A	100. B	134. A	168. D
33. C	67. B	101. D	135. D	169. A
34. C	68. B	102. C	136. A	170. C

171. D	218. A	265. D	312. C	359. D
172. B	219. C	266. A	313. C	360. D
173. A	220. A	267. D	314. D	361. C
174. E	221. B	268. B	315. D	362. C
175. B	222. A	269. B	316. A	363. C
176. A	223. B	270. D	317. C	364. B
177. D	224. C	271. B	318. D	365. C
178. B	225. A	272. C	319. E	366. C
179. A	226. B	273. B	320. C	367. D
180. C	227. E	274. C	321. D	368. C
181. A	228. C	275. C	322. E	369. C
182. C	229. B	276. B	323. A	370. D
183. C	230. D	277. D	324. E	371. D
184. B	231. D	278. B	325. D	372. E
185. D	232. A	279. C	326. A	373. E
186. A	233. B	280. C	327. A	374. B
187. B	234. C	281. C	328. A	375. C
188. B	235. D	282. C	329. B	376. C
189. B	236. D	283. C	330. D	377. C
190. B	237. B	284. D	331. A	378. D
191. C	238. A	285. A	332. A	379. B
192. A	239. C	286. D	333. C	380. C
193. C	240. A	287. B	334. C	381. B
194. C	241. B	288. B	335. C	382. B
195. A	242. D	289. B	336. D	383. B
196. A	243. C	290. A	337. A	384. B
197. B	244. D	291. B	338. D	385. A
198. B	245. C	292. A	339. C	386. C
199. D	246. B	293. B	340. C	387. B
200. D	247. A	294. C	341. D	388. D
201. A	248. B	295. E	342. A	389. D
202. C	249. D	296. C	343. C	390. C
203. D	250. D	297. D	344. B	391. E
204. B	251. B	298. D	345. C	392. C
205. B	252. A	299. B	346. B	393. E
206. D	253. A	300. D	347. C	394. D
207. C	254. B	301. A	348. D	395. B
208. C	255. B	302. E	349. C	396. A
209. B	256. A	303. A	350. A	397. B
210. A	257. E	304. C	351. C	398. A
211. A	258. D	305. B	352. C	399. E
212. E	259. D	306. B	353. D	400. A
213. A	260. A	307. C	354. A	401. B
214. C	261. C	308. D	355. C	402. C
215. C	262. C	309. D	356. E	403. D
216. B	263. C	310. D	357. C	404. C
217. C	264. B	311. A	358. C	405. C

406. E	424. B	442. C	460. E	478. B
407. B	425. C	443. A	461. A	479. A
408. E	426. C	444. B	462. D	480. C
409. B	427. B	445. C	463. B	481. B
410. C	428. E	446. E	464. C	482. D
411. C	429. D	447. A	465. B	483. A
412. C	430. C	448. E	466. D	484. A
413. D	431. B	449. A	467. A	485. D
414. C	432. C	450. C	468. A	486. D
415. C	433. E	451. C	469. B	487. C
416. B	434. C	452. B	470. C	488. C
417. A	435. D	453. C	471. C	489. A
418. C	436. C	454. C	472. A	490. A
419. D	437. A	455. D	473. D	491. A
420. C	438. B	456. A	474. B	492. D
421. B	439. B	457. A	475. C	493. C
422. B	440. D	458. C	476. D	494. C
423. D	441. A	459. D	477. B	

SAMPLE WRITTEN QUESTIONS

DOMAIN II: RECOGNITION, EVALUATION, AND ASSESSMENT

1. "Jumper's knee" is a lay term referring to
   A. Patellar chondromalacia.
   B. Osteochondritis dissecans.
   C. Tenosynovitis of the infrapatellar tendon.
   D. Osgood-Schlatter disease.
   E. Inflammation of the tibial tuberosity.

2. The step defect noted clinically would indicate that the athlete should be checked further by a physician for
   A. Spina bifida.
   B. Spondylolisthesis.
   C. Rheumatoid spondylitis.
   D. Degenerative disk disease.
   E. Osteoporosis.

3. When using a bag-valve-mask resuscitator, the most important factor is
   A. Opening the airway.
   B. The position of the person giving first aid.
   C. The rhythm or timing of breathing.
   D. Removing water from the lungs.
   E. The depth and sound of breathing.

4. The peroneal muscle group is often strained in conjunction with a/an
   A. Medial ankle sprain.
   B. Lateral ankle sprain.
   C. Anterior ankle sprain.
   D. Avulsion fracture of the ankle.
   E. Posterior ankle sprain.

5. It is dangerous to cause the victim to vomit in the event of
   A. Alcohol poisoning.
   B. Kerosene poisoning.
   C. Aspirin poisoning.
   D. Nicotine poisoning.
   E. Charcoal poisoning.

6. Severe hemorrhaging will eventually result in
   A. Shock.
   B. High blood pressure.
   C. Emesis.
   D. Hyperventilation.
   E. Hyperglycemia.

7. Winging of the scapula could result from injury to which one of the following nerves?
   A. Median
   B. Axillary
   C. Long thoracic
   D. Suprascapular
   E. Spinal accessory

8. When one wears an arm sling, the hand should
   A. Be lower than the elbow.
   B. Be even with the elbow.
   C. Be slightly higher than the elbow.
   D. Be covered by the sling.
   E. Remain clenched.

9. Closed-chest cardiac massage should be repeated
   A. 12 times per minute.
   B. 20 times per minute.
   C. 10 times per minute.
   D. In timing with artificial respiration procedure.
   E. Once in the field and then again in the hospital.

10. Back pain from muscle spasm is increased with active
    A. Extension.
    B. Flexion.
    C. Abduction.
    D. Rotation.
    E. Adduction.

11. Air as it exists in nature is approximately
    A. 5% oxygen.
    B. 10% oxygen.
    C. 15% oxygen.
    D. 20% oxygen.
    E. 49% oxygen.

12. Which of the following is not a joint-specific special test designed to assess an injury at the shoulder?
    A. Yergason's
    B. Speed's
    C. Phalen's
    D. Empty can
    E. Sulcus sign

13. All of the following are signs and symptoms of a Volkmann's contracture, except
    A. Pain in forearm.
    B. Passive extension of the fingers lessens the pain.
    C. Cessation of the brachial pulse.
    D. Cessation of the radial pulse.
    E. Coldness of the elbow, forearm, and hand.

14. In Caucasians, cyanosis causes the skin to turn
    A. White.
    B. Blue.
    C. Light red.
    D. Deep red.
    E. Pink.

15. A 16-year-old swimmer was diagnosed as having thoracic outlet syndrome. All of the following are possible causes except
    A. Constriction under the clavicle.
    B. Spastic anterior scalene muscle.
    C. Vertebrochondral rib.
    D. Tight smaller pectoral muscle.
    E. Traction injury to the long thoracic nerve.

16. A baseball player at bat is struck in the face by the ball. Which of the following signs or symptoms would suggest a fracture of the maxilla?
    A. Depression of the cheekbone and blurring of vision
    B. Facial pain and epistaxis
    C. Anterior open bite
    D. Malocclusion of the teeth and numbness of the cheek
    E. Hyphema and inability of the athlete to look upward

17. Hyperextension of the wrist causing pain in the anatomic "snuffbox" and decreased grip strength are indicative of which injury?
    A. Fracture of one of the metacarpals
    B. Fracture of the styloid process of the radius
    C. Fracture of the carpal navicular-scaphoid
    D. Fracture of the ulnar styloid process
    E. Colles' fracture

18. A quick and easy method to determine the shoulder's active range of motion is to have the athlete touch the opposite scapula from behind the head and/or up the center of the back. This test is commonly called
    A. Apley's scratch test.
    B. Yergason's test.
    C. Drop arm test.
    D. Apprehension test.
    E. Crossover test.

19. Which bone lies directly proximal to the first metacarpal?
    A. Trapezoid
    B. Pisiform
    C. Trapezium
    D. Navicular
    E. Lunate

20. The rapid improvement with rest of the clinical symptoms of step defect, flattening of the lumbar spine, and tight hamstrings suggests which of the following pathologies?
    A. Spina bifida
    B. Degenerative disk
    C. Spondylolisthesis
    D. Rheumatoid spondylitis
    E. Congenital disease

21. A simple partial epileptic seizure is characterized by
    A. A catatonic state.
    B. A brief bout of uncontrolled shaking of the limbs on one side of the body and no loss of consciousness.
    C. A brief bout of uncontrolled shaking of the limbs and no loss of consciousness.
    D. A brief bout of uncontrolled shaking of the limbs with a loss of consciousness.
    E. Total body convulsions and a loss of consciousness.

22. When using the SOAP format, the information detailing what the patient tells the athletic trainer about the injury relative to the history or the pain felt should be recorded in the
    A. "S" section.
    B. "O" section.
    C. "A" section.
    D. "P" section
    E. Appendix section because it is only ancillary information.

23. An apprehension test for the knee is performed to evaluate
    A. Chondromalacia.
    B. Jumper's knee.
    C. Patellar-femoral stress syndrome.
    D. Patellar instability.
    E. Patellar osteochondritis.

24. An athlete comes into the athletic training room and displays the following signs and symptoms: tender lymph nodes, tender left side, low-grade fever, and sore throat. The athlete may have
    A. Mononucleosis.
    B. Strep throat.
    C. Appendicitis.
    D. Pneumonia.
    E. Influenza.

25. A male athlete comes to the athletic trainer complaining of painful urination and pus discharge from the genitals and confides that he had unprotected sexual contact approximately 1 week earlier. Based on his symptoms, what should the athletic trainer suspect is the athlete's immediate problem?
    A. Tinea capitis
    B. Gonorrhea
    C. Acquired immunodeficiency syndrome
    D. Impetigo contagiosa
    E. Hepatitis

26. What would be a complication of a medial ankle sprain?
    A. Avulsion fracture
    B. Chondromalacia
    C. Myositis ossificans traumatica
    D. Osgood-Schlatter disease
    E. Hyphema.

27. An athlete has been diagnosed as having myositis ossificans. Which of the following is a factor contributing to the condition?
    A. Isometric exercise
    B. Passive stretching
    C. Intramuscular bleeding
    D. Weight-bearing activity
    E. High-volt-pulsed stimulation

28. During your examination, you have the athlete make a fist and extend the wrist against resistance while stabilizing the forearm. If you elicit pain at the lateral epicondyle of the athlete's elbow, which of the following conditions would you suspect?
    A. Olecranon bursitis
    B. Lateral epicondylitis
    C. Occlusion of the brachial artery
    D. Neuroma of the ulnar nerve
    E. Triceps tendinitis

29. Which of the following would not be considered a postconcussion symptom?
    A. Headache
    B. Steady gait
    C. Behavior changes
    D. Fatigue
    E. Tinnitus

30. Factors contributing to repeated eruption of herpes type II lesions involve all of the following except
    A. Fatigue.
    B. Psychological stress.
    C. Sexual activity.
    D. Reinfection.
    E. Poor nutrition.

31. Which sign is inconsistent with hypovolemic shock?
    A. Systolic blood pressure below 100 mmHg
    B. Weak radial pulse
    C. Pulse rate above 110 beats per minute
    D. Warm, dry skin
    E. Rapid, shallow breathing

32. In a contusion of the medial epicondyle of the humerus, the nerve most likely to be damaged is the
    A. Median.
    B. Radial.
    C. Brachial.
    D. Ulnar.
    E. Musculocutaneous.

33. Postconcussion syndrome symptoms include which three domains?
    A. Somatic, affective, cognitive
    B. Affective, cognitive, mental

    C. Cognitive, somatic, effective
    D. Somatic, affective, depressive
    E. Effective, cognitive, affective

34. In regard to dispensing medications, an athletic trainer should
    A. Provide only over-the-counter medication to the athlete.
    B. Buy only recognized nongeneric medications.
    C. Insist that the physician prescribe and dispense all medications.
    D. Keep all medications under lock and key in the athletic trainer's office.
    E. Dispense all medications from the athletic trainer's office.

35. A basketball player sustains trauma to the eye that causes bleeding into the anterior chamber. This injury is classified as a/an
    A. Hyphema.
    B. Corneal abrasion.
    C. Subconjunctival hematoma.
    D. Diplopia.
    E. Detached retina.

36. Which orthopedic special test is performed by externally rotating the athlete's arm as he or she resists while pulling downward on his or her elbow?
    A. McMurray's test
    B. Yergason's test
    C. Reduction click test
    D. Apley's compression distraction test
    E. Tinel's sign

37. The way to determine entrapment of the inferior muscle of the eye as a result of a blowout fracture is to have the person
    A. Move his or her eyes to the right.
    B. Move his or her eyes to the left.
    C. Move his or her eyes up.
    D. Move his or her eyes down.
    E. Close his or her eyes.

38. Which orthopedic special test is used with a suspected torn meniscus and is performed with the athlete in a prone position and leg flexed to 90 degrees?
    A. McMurray's test
    B. Yergason's test
    C. Reduction click test

D. Apley's compression distraction test

E. Tinel's sign

39. In which of the following conditions is tinnitus a characteristic sign?
    A. Tenosynovitis
    B. Hypothermia
    C. Hyperthermia
    D. Cerebral concussion
    E. Myositis ossificans

40. Injury to the spleen often results in referred pain in the upper left quadrant. This event is also referred to as
    A. Tinel's sign.
    B. Kehr's sign.
    C. Battle's sign.
    D. Murphy's sign.
    E. Romberg's sign.

41. Metatarsalgia under the second metatarsal head could be caused by which of the following conditions?
    A. Hammer toes
    B. Hallux valgus
    C. Foot pronation
    D. Foot supination
    E. Bunionette

42. During a gymnastics meet, an athlete falls from the balance beam, injuring her right shoulder. Palpation reveals a posterior displacement of the head of the humerus. The athlete's arm is abducted approximately 45 degrees, and any movement results in severe pain. The decision is made to splint the arm as it was found using pillows and cravats. Which of the following should be assessed before and after the splint is applied?
    A. Blood pressure in the injured arm
    B. Heart rate, rhythm, and strength
    C. Distal neurovascular and circulatory functions
    D. Respiratory rate, rhythm, and depth
    E. Strength of the forearm muscles

43. Inverting and dorsiflexing the ankle against resistance is a test used to assess the
    A. Posterior tibial muscle.
    B. Peroneal muscle.
    C. Anterior tibial muscle.
    D. Long muscle of the great toe.
    E. Anterior talofibular.

44. Inverting and plantar flexing the ankle against resistance is a test used to assess the
    A. Posterior tibial muscle.
    B. Peroneal muscle.
    C. Anterior tibial muscle.
    D. Long muscle of the great toe.
    E. Anterior talofibular muscle/ligament.

45. The best way to determine the pulse rate of an athlete who has a weak pulse is to palpate the
    _____ artery.
    A. Foot's dorsal
    B. Subclavian
    C. Vertebral
    D. Carotid
    E. Radial

46. The most reliable examinations in evaluating nerve involvement in back trauma are
    A. Stress tests.
    B. Functional tests.
    C. Reflex tests.
    D. Sensory tests.
    E. Neuromuscular tests.

47. The eating disorder bulimia is characterized by all of the following signs except
    A. Abuse of laxatives or diuretics.
    B. Increased incidence of caries.
    C. Underachieving.
    D. Distorted body image.
    E. Short periods of starvation.

48. The individual who is ultimately responsible for determining the athlete's medical ability to return to competition is the
    A. Physician.
    B. Athletic trainer.
    C. Parent.
    D. Coach.
    E. Athletic director.

49. Immature stress fractures are **best** visualized through which diagnostic technique?
    A. Bone scan
    B. Stress x-rays
    C. Ultrasound
    D. Arthrogram
    E. Tomograms

50. Following trauma, the initial response of a blood vessel is
    A. Margination followed by vasoconstriction.
    B. Transient vasodilation followed by vasoconstriction.
    C. Continual vasoconstriction.
    D. Transient vasoconstriction followed by vasodilation.
    E. Pavementing.

51. This type of overuse syndrome is characterized by tenderness at the point of attachment and sharp pain in the area of the medial longitudinal arch; pain increases with weight bearing, especially when the athlete steps out of bed in the morning.
    A. Morton's neuroma
    B. Achilles tendinitis
    C. Retrocalcaneal bursitis
    D. Sesamoiditis
    E. Plantar fasciitis

52. Generally speaking, "shin splints" is a painful condition associated with stress that pulls the anterior and posterior tibial muscles away from the
    A. Interosseus membrane.
    B. Periosteal origin.
    C. Metatarsals.
    D. Tibial tuberosity.
    E. Calcaneus.

53. An axial compression fracture in football players **most** commonly occurs when the neck is in which position?
    A. Partial flexion
    B. Hyperextension
    C. Lateral flexion
    D. Partial extension
    E. Rotation

54. When evaluating a knee joint injury, an important anatomic consideration for a possible meniscal injury is the fact that the
    A. Medial and lateral menisci are attached to their respective collateral ligaments and become distorted during tibial rotation.
    B. Medial and lateral menisci are torn when the ligaments are forced into extreme rotation.
    C. The medial meniscus is attached to the medial collateral ligament and becomes distorted during tibial rotation.
    D. The lateral meniscus is attached to the lateral collateral ligament and becomes distorted during tibial rotation.
    E. Medial and lateral menisci are not attached to ligaments and are free to move during tibial rotation.

55. When performing one-person cardiopulmonary respiration, the proper compression to breath ratio is
    A. 5:1.
    B. 5:2.
    C. 15:1.
    D. 15:2.
    E. 2:15.

56. Which of the following groups of muscles insert into the medial aspect of the tibia just distal to the medial condyle?
    A. Medial vastus, gracilis, and semimembranous
    B. Semitendinous, sartorius, and medial vastus
    C. Biceps muscle of the thigh, semitendinous, and femoral
    D. Sartorius, gracilis, and semitendinous
    E. Sartorius, gracilis, and semimembranous

57. Which of the following signs and symptoms are associated with a gradual onset of a subdural hematoma?
    A. Raccoon eyes
    B. Hematuria
    C. Increased pulse rate
    D. Deterioration of consciousness
    E. Epistaxis

58. Lumbar hyperlordosis is an abnormal spinal curve best described as
    A. A convex curve of the upper thorax.
    B. A concave curve of the lumbar area.
    C. A lateral curve often with rotation.
    D. A concave curve of the cervical area.
    E. A lateral curve of the cervical area.

59. Which of the following is a sign or symptom of traumatic shock?
    A. Decreased pulse rate
    B. Decreased blood pressure
    C. Tinnitus
    D. Nystagmus
    E. Decreased respiratory rate

60. Which one of the following tests is used to detect possible rotator cuff tears?
    A. McMurray's
    B. Lachman
    C. Yergason's
    D. Drop arm
    E. Apprehension

61. Early signs of internal bleeding include
    A. Weak, slow pulse.
    B. Restlessness, anxiety, and thirst.
    C. Sweating and fever.
    D. Cold and clammy skin.
    E. Unequal pupils.

62. During the observation-inspection phase of injury assessment, it is important for the athletic trainer to gather which of the following pieces of information.
    A. The severity of pain
    B. The presence of crepitation
    C. The amount of swelling or ecchymosis
    D. The presence of paresthesia
    E. The type of activity that caused the pain

63. The phase of a grand mal seizure that may alert an individual with epilepsy to an oncoming attack is the
    A. Aura stage.
    B. Clonic stage.
    C. Postictal stage.
    D. Status stage.
    E. Tonic-clonic stage.

64. Rotation of the spine in the transverse plane is **greatest** at the
    A. Thoracic vertebrae.
    B. Cervical vertebrae.
    C. Thoracolumbar junction.
    D. Lumbar vertebrae.
    E. Lumbosacral junction.

65. The Allen's test at the shoulder involves which muscle specifically?
    A. Sternocleidomastoid
    B. Smaller pectoral
    C. Greater pectoral
    D. Anterior scalene
    E. Latissimus dorsi

66. Which of the following tissues has the least likelihood of regenerating?
    A. Skin
    B. Muscle
    C. Bone
    D. Peripheral nervous system
    E. Central nervous system

67. Back injuries can be described as falling into one of three categories. These are
    A. Sprain/strain, fracture, ruptured disk.
    B. Sprain, strain, mechanical problems.
    C. Sprain/strain, mechanical problems, ruptured disk.
    D. Mechanical problems, spondylosis, ruptured disk.
    E. Sprain/strain, fracture, mechanical problem.

68. Which is not a sign of a basilar skull fracture?
    A. Battle's sign
    B. Hemotympanum
    C. Otorrhea
    D. Rales
    E. Raccoon eyes

69. Pale skin color indicates which of the following conditions?
    A. High blood pressure
    B. Poisoning
    C. Asphyxia
    D. Heat stroke
    E. Shock

70. All of the following can be signs of internal bleeding **except**
    A. Increased blood pressure.
    B. Weak, rapid pulse.
    C. Abdominal rigidity.
    D. Blood in the urine, stool, or vomit.
    E. Bleeding from the ears.

71. The inversion ankle sprain is more common than the eversion ankle injury because
    A. Bony stability is greater on the lateral side.
    B. Muscles that evert the ankle are stronger than invertors.
    C. Bony stability is greater on the medial side.
    D. The deltoid ligament is shorter than the lateral ligaments are.
    E. The lateral ligament complex is much stronger.

72. The shoulder is often subjected to direct blows. This may cause a contusion or it may result in an acromioclavicular (AC) separation. Which of the following distinguishes a mild separation from a contusion?
    A. Painful to touch opposite shoulder with hand of injured part
    B. Point tenderness of AC joint area
    C. Swelling
    D. Laxity of AC joint when pressure is put on middle third of the clavicle
    E. Redness and pain in the area

73. Which type of fracture would most likely cause a pneumothorax?
    A. Direct
    B. Indirect
    C. Open
    D. Closed
    E. Hairline

74. A blow to the lateral side of the knee puts what kind of stress on the knee?
    A. Valgus
    B. Varus
    C. Internal rotation
    D. Lateral
    E. External rotation

75. The dislocation of a joint also will cause a
    A. Severe strain.
    B. Fracture.
    C. Severe sprain.
    D. Subluxation.
    E. Break.

76. A scraping of the skin is called a/an
    A. Incision.
    B. Abrasion.
    C. Laceration.
    D. Suture.
    E. Tear.

77. Symptoms of a stress injury are
    A. Specific trauma, swelling, discoloration, pain.
    B. No specific trauma, inflammation, pain.
    C. Specific trauma, inflammation, pain.
    D. No specific trauma, deformity, pain.
    E. Specific trauma, discoloration, inflammation.

78. Soft corns are found
    A. On the ball of the foot.
    B. On bony prominences of the foot.
    C. Between the toes.
    D. On top of the toes.
    E. Under the toenails.

79. The anterior and posterior drawer tests for the knee are designed to stress which of the following?
    A. Medial collateral ligaments
    B. Cruciate ligaments
    C. Cartilage
    D. Hamstrings
    E. Lateral collateral ligaments

80. A hip pointer is a
    A. Muscle strain occurring at the iliac crest.
    B. Contusion to the iliac crest.
    C. Fracture of the iliac crest.
    D. Prominent iliac crest.
    E. Muscle sprain occurring at the iliac crest.

81. Softening of the back of the patella from a persistent inflammatory condition is called
    A. Osgood-Schlatter disease.
    B. Chondromalacia.
    C. Jumper's knee.
    D. Patellar tendonitis.
    E. Patellar sprain.

82. Mallet finger is a/an
    A. Congenital deformity.
    B. Extensor tendonitis of the distal phalanx.
    C. Avulsion of the extensor tendon of the distal phalanx.
    D. Fracture of the distal phalanx.
    E. Sprain of the distal phalanx.

83. The unhappy triad injury involves which three structures?
    A. Medial collateral ligament, medial meniscus, posterior cruciate ligament
    B. Medial collateral ligament, medial meniscus, anterior cruciate ligament
    C. Lateral collateral ligament, biceps muscle of the thigh, lateral meniscus
    D. Gracilis muscle, hamstring muscles, medial collateral ligament
    E. Lateral collateral ligament, medial collateral ligament, posterior cruciate ligament

84. The mechanism of injury for a lateral ankle sprain is usually
    A. Eversion.
    B. Inversion.
    C. Eversion, torsion.
    D. Inversion, plantar flexion.
    E. External rotation.

85. Morton's neuroma
    A. Means that the second toe is longer than the first.
    B. Is found between the third and fourth metatarsal.
    C. Is found behind the knee.
    D. Is a vascular problem.
    E. Is a neuromuscular disease.

86. The common mechanism of injury for a shoulder dislocation is
    A. A fall on an outstretched arm.
    B. The arm forced in abduction and external rotation.
    C. A direct blow to the acromioclavicular joint.
    D. The arm forced in horizontal adduction and external rotation.
    E. The arm forced in internal rotation and abduction.

87. Testing an athlete suspected of having a concussion by having the athlete stand with feet together, arms at side, and eyes closed is known as the
    A. Romberg test.
    B. Pupil test.
    C. Eye, hand, foot test.
    D. Tandem gait test.
    E. Heal to shin test.

88. The local reaction of the body tissues to an irritant is called
    A. Abrasives.
    B. Stenosity.
    C. Inflammation.
    D. Irritability.
    E. Pain recognition.

89. By definition a sprain is
    A. Damage to the musculotendinous unit.
    B. Damage to any soft tissue structures.
    C. Damage to the vascular structures.
    D. Damage to the ligamentous structures.
    E. Damage to the integrity of the bone.

90. Which of the following would be found during palpation?
    A. Point tenderness
    B. Ecchymosis
    C. Dyspnea
    D. Allergies
    E. Stridor

91. All of these are symptoms of concussion except
    A. Loss of balance.
    B. Confusion.
    C. Extreme hunger.
    D. Headache.
    E. Disturbance in vision.

92. Stress testing is basically
    A. Testing muscle function through a complete range of motion.
    B. Testing ligament stability.
    C. Allowing athletes to participate in activity.
    D. Testing an athlete's endurance.
    E. Testing tendon stability.

93. A lacrosse player is hit on the medial right elbow with a lacrosse stick and reports to you with pain and tingling in the little and ring fingers. Grip strength and sensations are normal for the other fingers and thumb. What structure was irritated?
    A. Median nerve
    B. Radian nerve
    C. Musculocutaneous nerve
    D. Brachial plexus
    E. Ulnar nerve

94. To isolate the brachial muscle for resisted range of motion for extension and flexion of the elbow, the forearm should be in what position?
    A. The forearm should be supinated.
    B. The forearm should be pronated.
    C. The forearm should be in the neutral position.
    D. The forearm should be extended.
    E. The forearm should be flexed.

95. As it relates to a knee evaluation, which is not a bony landmark of the knee?
    A. Fibula
    B. Adductor tubercle
    C. Femoral epicondyle
    D. Trochanter
    E. Lateral tibial condyle.

96. The distraction test helps distinguish between
    A. Meniscal tears and hamstring strain.
    B. Hamstring strain and ligamentous sprain.
    C. Meniscal tears and ligamentous sprain.
    D. Cruciate ligament sprain and collateral ligament sprain.
    E. Meniscal tears and plica syndrome.

97. The "screw home motion" or locking of the knee occurs at complete extension. At this point what happens to the tibia?
    A. It rotates internally.
    B. It rotates externally.
    C. It adducts.
    D. It abducts.
    E. Nothing.

98. Which of the following tests cranial nerve II?
    A. Lateral and vertical gaze
    B. Double simultaneous stimulation of the trigeminal nerve
    C. Symmetric smile
    D. Visual acuity
    E. Pupil reaction to light

99. Which is not true about a Baker's cyst?
    A. Painless mobile swelling
    B. Often malignant
    C. Distention of the gastrocnemius muscle bursa or the semimembranous bursa
    D. Found in popliteal fossa
    E. Often benign

100. The lateral meniscus is attached to the
    A. Head of the fibula.
    B. Biceps tendon.
    C. Plantar muscle.
    D. Popliteal muscle.
    E. Patella.

101. Ecchymosis around the mastoid process, as an indication of a basilar skull fracture, is referred to as
    A. Tinel's sign
    B. Kehr's sign
    C. Battle's sign
    D. Murphy's sign
    E. Romberg's sign

102. Laxity after valgus stress to the knee, a positive anterior drawer test, and tenderness along the medial joint line are symptoms associated with
    A. Medial collateral ligament sprain.
    B. Lateral collateral ligament sprain.
    C. Anterior cruciate ligament sprain.
    D. Injury to the medial meniscus.
    E. The unhappy triad.

103. The classic mechanism of injury for a medial collateral ligament is
    A. Valgus stress, internal rotation of thigh.
    B. Valgus stress, internal rotation of leg.
    C. Valgus stress, external rotation of thigh.
    D. External rotation of leg.
    E. Varus stress.

104. Pes planus is
    A. Abnormally high arch.
    B. Plantar flexion.
    C. Absence of medial longitudinal arch.
    D. Excessive hindfoot varus.
    E. Extreme lateral rotation.

105. A positive drawer test in the ankle indicates loss of integrity of which ligament?
    A. Anterior talofibular
    B. Calcaneofibular
    C. Deltoid
    D. Tibiofibular
    E. Posterior tibial

106. Scoliosis is an abnormal spinal curve best described as a
    A. Convex curve of the upper thorax.
    B. Concave curve of the lumbar area.
    C. Lateral curve often with rotation.
    D. Concave curve of the cervical area.
    E. Lateral curve of the cervical area.

107. What special test for the elbow tests the integrity of the radial collateral ligament, the annular ligament, the accessory lateral collateral ligament, and the lateral ulnar collateral ligament?
    A. Varus stress test
    B. Valgus stress test
    C. Posterolateral rotatory instability test
    D. Gravity stress test
    E. Valgus extension overload test

108. When the calcaneus is forced into extreme eversion, the talus is rotated and forced against the distal ends of the tibia and fibula, causing the tibiofibular ligament to rupture. This injury is called
    A. Pott's fracture.
    B. Spread mortise.
    C. Avulsion fracture.
    D. Anterior compartment syndrome.
    E. Maiolo syndrome.

109. A concussion is defined as a/an
    A. Contusion, usually resulting in hemorrhage.
    B. Bruise of the brain.
    C. Intracranial hemorrhage.
    D. Stroke.
    E. Headache lasting longer than 3 days.

110. Symptoms of a first-degree concussion include
    A. Intracranial hemorrhage.
    B. Loss of consciousness.
    C. Tinnitus.
    D. Paralysis.
    E. Amnesia.

111. When the brain loses autoregulation of its blood supply, vascular engorgement within the cranium results, which in turn leads to herniation either of the medial surface of the temporal lobe or lobes below the tentorium or of the cerebellar tonsils through the foramen magnum. This condition, which leads to rapid brainstem failure within 2 to 5 minutes, is called
    A. Antegrade amnesia.
    B. Transient ischemic attack.
    C. Skull fracture.
    D. Cerebral concussion.
    E. Second impact syndrome.

112. Which muscle in the rotator cuff is not palpable?
    A. Supraspinous
    B. Infraspinous
    C. Teres minor
    D. Subscapular
    E. Biceps

113. Which ligament of the shoulder is not usually injured in an acromioclavicular separation?
    A. Capsular
    B. Trapezoid
    C. Coracoacromial
    D. Coronoid
    E. Rotator cuff

114. A collection of a thick fluid within a tendinous sheath or joint capsule is called
    A. Erb's palsy.
    B. Ganglion cyst.
    C. Bursa.
    D. Paronychia.
    E. Hill-Sachs lesion.

115. Which of the following terms are not matched correctly?
    A. Anesthesia: absence of sensation
    B. Hypoesthesia: decreased sensation
    C. Paresthesia: abnormal sensation
    D. Megesthesia: increased sensation
    E. Hypesthesia: increased sensation

116. Which is not true for the apprehension test for anterior glenohumeral laxity?
    A. The glenohumeral joint is abducted to 90 degrees; the elbow is flexed at 90 degrees.
    B. One should test the uninvolved side first.
    C. It tests for anterior capsule and/or glenoid labrum compromise.
    D. It should be avoided when it is apparent that a glenohumeral joint dislocation has occurred.
    E. It should be performed late in the evaluation because of the pain it may cause the athlete.

117. The brachial plexus is made up of nerves that are derived from which of the following nerve roots?
    A. C-2 through C-6
    B. C-3 through C-7
    C. C-4 through C-8
    D. C-5 through T-1
    E. C-5 through T-3

118. A grade-1 concussion according to the Colorado scale is
    A. No loss of consciousness, confusion, no amnesia.
    B. Loss of consciousness for less than 5 minutes, amnesia, vertigo.
    C. Momentary loss of consciousness, tinnitis, dazed appearance.
    D. No loss of consciousness, confusion, amnesia.
    E. No loss of consciousness, post-traumatic amnesia for less than 30 minutes, dazed appearance.

119. An accentuated lordosis is usually related to
    A. Tight hip flexor muscles and weak abdominal muscles.
    B. Tight gluteal muscles and weak abdominal muscles.
    C. Tight dorsal spine and weak hip flexor muscles.
    D. Tight abdominal muscles and weak gluteal muscles.
    E. Tight abdominal muscles and weak hip flexor muscles.

120. Pain appearing to emanate from the sacroiliac joint may actually come from a
    A. Fractured coccyx.
    B. Sciatic irritation.
    C. Trochanteric bursitis.
    D. Piriform strain.
    E. Dislocation.

121. The carpal tunnel is located in the
    A. Knee.
    B. Ankle.
    C. Anterior compartment of the wrist.
    D. Posterior compartment of the wrist.
    E. Hand.

122. The carpal tunnel is formed by the attachment of the volar ligament to the
    A. Phalanges.
    B. Metacarpals.
    C. Carpal bones.
    D. Radial epicondyle.
    E. Ulnar epicondyle.

123. Carpal tunnel syndrome is a result of
    A. Contusion and compression of the flexor tendons.
    B. Constriction of the carpal tunnel, putting pressure on the median nerve.
    C. Effusion of the carpal bones.
    D. An avulsion of the volar ligament at its attachment to the metacarpals.
    E. Contusion to the anterior compartment of the wrist.

124. A sign of a carpal tunnel syndrome injury is tingling of the
    A. Tip of the thumb.
    B. Tips of the toes.
    C. Tips of the long fingers.
    D. The wrist.
    E. The elbow.

125. A Colles' fracture occurs at the
    A. Proximal part of the radius and/or ulna.
    B. Distal part of the radius and/or ulna.
    C. Lower leg.
    D. Midportion of the ulna.
    E. Midportion of the radius.

126. The navicular bone is located under the anatomic "snuff box" on the
    A. Radial aspect of the wrist.
    B. Palmar aspect of the wrist.
    C. Ulnar aspect of the wrist.
    D. Dorsal aspect of the wrist.
    E. Posterior aspect of the wrist.

127. A navicular fracture is difficult to evaluate because
    A. The navicular bone is too dense for x-rays to pass through.
    B. A fracture line may not show on x-rays for several weeks.
    C. The wrist cannot be stabilized because of a chronic or acute irritation of the proximal radial condyle.
    D. It may take several months for a fracture line to show on x-rays.
    E. The navicular bone is too small to be seen by x-ray.

128. What is the term used to describe the intense pain experienced by a patient when an examiner presses into his or her abdomen and then quickly releases?
    A. Tenderness
    B. Bounding tenderness
    C. Reflex pain
    D. Rebound phenomenon
    E. Rebound tenderness

129. Mallet finger is most common in
    A. Golf.
    B. Tennis.
    C. Handball.
    D. Baseball.
    E. Water polo.

130. A football player whose position on the team is tight end comes into the athletic training room after a game, walking with his torso bent to the right. He reports sustaining a blow to his right lower back during a play. He is experiencing pain throughout the right side of the back and in the groin. The athletic trainer notices muscle spasms in the athlete's back after removal of the player's shirt. The athletic trainer suspects a kidney contusion. What should the athletic trainer have the athlete watch for and report?
    A. Increased hunger
    B. Hematuria
    C. Dyspnea
    D. Vertigo
    E. Hemarthrosis

131. Which is a special test for biceps tendinitis?
    A. Distraction test
    B. Empty can test
    C. Speed's test
    D. Apprehension test
    E. Drop arm test

132. What is the name of the special test that assesses for carpal tunnel syndrome?
    A. Bunnel-Littler test
    B. Speed's test
    C. Adson's test
    D. Phalen's test
    E. Pinch test

133. In dark-skinned people, cyanosis is best seen by observing the
    A. Eyes.
    B. Lips and abdomen.
    C. Tongue and nail beds.
    D. Earlobes.
    E. Pupils.

134. To assess possible cervical nerve root trauma, the athletic trainer should check
    A. Neck flexion and extension.
    B. Unilateral sensory and motor function in the upper extremities.
    C. Bilateral sensory and motor function in the upper extremities.
    D. Resisted neck range of motion.
    E. Neck rotation left and right.

135. Unilateral change in pupil size may be found as a sign of head injury. What other condition might present with the same sign?
    A. Anisocoria
    B. Poisoning
    C. Drug overdose
    D. Heat exhaustion
    E. Shock

136. A condition that affects the ability to dorsiflex and invert the ankle and foot is
    A. Calcaneal apophysitis.
    B. Shin splints.
    C. Tibial muscle posterior strain.
    D. Drop foot.
    E. Plantar muscle rupture.

137. Which test elicits pain when a nerve is tapped, possibly indicating a neuroma?
    A. McMurray's test
    B. Yergason's test
    C. Reduction click test
    D. Apley's compression distraction test
    E. Tinel's sign

138. All of the following are signs or symptoms of acute trauma to the abdomen except
    A. Rigidity.
    B. Tenderness.
    C. Guarding.
    D. Rebound tenderness.
    E. Bowel sounds.

139. A test to specifically identify posterior medial meniscal tears is
    A. McMurray's test.
    B. Yergason's test.
    C. Reduction click test.
    D. Apley's compression distraction test.
    E. Tinel's sign.

140. What is another name for stenosing tenosynovitis of dorsal carpal tunnel #1?
    A. Guyon's disease
    B. Gamekeeper's thumb
    C. de Quervain's disease
    D. Swan neck deformity
    E. Johnson's disease

141. What procedure is applied as a remedy for patients having a locked knee due to a torn, dislocated, or "heaped up" meniscus?
    A. McMurray's test
    B. Yergason's test
    C. Reduction click test
    D. Apley's compression distraction test
    E. Tinel's sign

142. Generally speaking, the blister cover should not be removed because
    A. It prevents infection and enlargement of the wound, and the wound heals faster.
    B. The athlete feels better immediately, and it prevents infection and helps visual observation.
    C. It prevents additional skin from tearing and fights fungus.
    D. It prevents enlargement, fights fungus, and allows the wound to heal faster.
    E. It keeps moisture out, prevents infection, and allows the wound to heal faster.

143. Tendonitis on the dorsal surface of the foot can be protected by
    A. Bridging with felt pads.
    B. Taping tightly.
    C. Exercising.
    D. Bridging with a sponge pad.
    E. Bridging with a gauze pad.

144. A shoulder separation is the common term for a disturbance of the articular junction of the
    A. Sternoclavicular joint.
    B. Acromioclavicular joint.
    C. Glenohumeral joint.
    D. Radioulnar joint.
    E. Scapulothoracic articulation.

145. The following are all tests for coordination except
    A. Rapid alternating movements.
    B. Heel to shin.
    C. Finger to nose.
    D. Knee drift.
    E. Tandem gait.

146. A common fracture that often occurs in the fifth metatarsal is a
    A. Jones fracture.
    B. Parade fracture.
    C. Pressure fracture.
    D. Stein-Haus fracture.
    E. Hairline fracture.

147. Which test evaluates thoracic outlet syndrome, in which the smaller pectoral muscle is compressing the neurovascular bundle?
    A. Adson's test
    B. Drop arm test
    C. Empty can test
    D. Allen's test
    E. Finkelstein's test

148. When there is pain on both sides of the ankle, one side might be sprained and the other might
    A. Have a contusion to the articular surfaces of the joint.
    B. Have most of the vascular damage.
    C. Be inflamed with bursitis.
    D. Be fractured.
    E. Have compression to the ligaments and tendons.

149. When an athlete has a medial ankle sprain, the athletic trainer should also suspect
    A. An avulsion fracture.
    B. A torn cartilage.
    C. A ruptured joint capsule.
    D. An extreme amount of swelling.
    E. Vascular damage.

150. Hemorrhage around an ankle sprain is indicative of
    A. The severity of the sprain.
    B. A corresponding strain.
    C. The amount of vascular damage.
    D. The amount of swelling.
    E. A torn cartilage.

151. How many times per minute should you repeat mouth-to-mouth artificial respiration?
    A. 5–7
    B. 12–14
    C. 17–19
    D. 22–24
    E. 25–30

152. The tibiofibular or transverse ligament injury poses a greater problem than usual ankle sprains because of the possibility of a/an
    A. Avulsion fracture.
    B. Spread mortise.

C. Complete rupture.

D. March or fatigue fracture.

E. Parade fracture.

153. Which of the following would not be a mechanism of a lateral ankle sprain?

    A. Inversion

    B. Eversion

    C. Plantar flexion

    D. Torsion

    E. Supination

154. Which of the following would not be included in immediate treatment for ankle sprains?

    A. I.C.E.

    B. Support

    C. Crutches

    D. Whirlpool

    E. Analgesics

155. While not wearing a helmet, a baseball player is hit in the head with a baseball. The player is stunned but walks off the field without assistance. After getting to the dugout, the player experiences a severe headache and deterioration to unconsciousness. What is happening to this athlete?

    A. Epidural hematoma

    B. Subarachnoid hematoma

    C. Postconcussive symptom

    D. Subdural hematoma

    E. Chronic brain injuries

156. Most ankle injuries occur to the

    A. Anterior aspect of the ankle.

    B. Lateral aspect of the ankle.

    C. Posterior aspect of the ankle.

    D. Medial aspect of the ankle.

    E. Superior aspect of the ankle.

157. Identify the radiological technique that most clearly identifies soft-tissue pathology.

    A. Bone scan

    B. Stress radiography

    C. Arthrography

    D. Electromyography

    E. Magnetic resonance imagery (MRI)

158. Injuries to the thigh in athletics generally are either

    A. Sprains or strains.

    B. Sprains or contusions.

    C. Strains or contusions.

    D. Fractures or strains.

    E. Fractures or contusions.

159. Injuries involving excessive vascular damage in and around the thigh always create a concern about

    A. Myositis ossificans.

    B. Blood clots.

    C. Pigmentation.

    D. Aspiration.

    E. Fat emboli.

160. Chondromalacia is

    A. A breakdown of cartilaginous tissue.

    B. An inflammation of the tibial tuberosity.

    C. A tearing of the meniscus.

    D. A softening of the articular cartilage.

    E. Friction between the patella and the tibial tuberosity.

161. The area in athletes that chondromalacia most often affects is the

    A. Epiphyseal line.

    B. Patella.

    C. Quadriceps.

    D. Tibial tuberosity.

    E. Femur.

162. During the course of a contest, two athletes collide. As a result, one of the athletes experiences a contralateral extension of the neck and head while the involved shoulder is thrust posteriorly. The athlete comes off of the field holding the injured arm and complaining of an extreme burning sensation, numbness, and weakness of the arm. What type of injury has this athlete sustained?

    A. Bursitis

    B. Brachial plexus injury

    C. Acromioclavicular separation

    D. Rotator cuff strain

    E. Ulnar fracture

163. Osteochondritis dissecans is

    A. Bone cartilage inflammation.

    B. Fracture lines in the tibial tuberosity.

    C. Joint obstructions.

    D. Interference of epiphysis.

    E. Inflammation of the tibial tuberosity.

164. The medial meniscus is often damaged in conjunction with medial collateral ligament injuries because
    A. It is large and bulky.
    B. It atrophies so rapidly.
    C. The two are anatomically attached.
    D. The fibular attachment is weak.
    E. The fibular attachment is soft.

165. Osgood-Schlatter disease in adolescence is often associated with
    A. Contact.
    B. Rapid growth.
    C. Trauma.
    D. Bacteria.
    E. Fracture.

166. A positive anterior drawer sign is indicative of
    A. Medial collateral ligament damage.
    B. Medial meniscus damage.
    C. Anterior cruciate damage.
    D. Popliteal damage.
    E. Posterior cruciate damage.

167. Osteochondral fracture is most common in the
    A. Ankle.
    B. Knee.
    C. Hip.
    D. Shoulder.
    E. Pelvis.

168. Which of the symptoms below is not a symptom of shock?
    A. Clammy skin
    B. Dilated pupils
    C. Strong, slow pulse
    D. Profuse sweating
    E. Hyperventilation

169. Apply a valgus stress to the medial side of the knee joint while you rotate the leg externally. While maintaining the valgus stress and external rotation, slowly extend the leg and palpate the medial joint line. This process describes
    A. McMurray's test.
    B. Yergason's test.
    C. Reduction click test.
    D. Apley's compression distraction test.
    E. Tinel's sign.

170. A separated shoulder is a/an
    A. Sternoclavicular sprain.
    B. Sternoclavicular strain.
    C. Acromioclavicular sprain.
    D. Acromioclavicular strain.
    E. Glenohumeral strain.

171. Which of the following signs of symptoms is associated with insulin shock?
    A. Dry mucous lining of the mouth
    B. Labored breathing
    C. Fruity smelling breath
    D. Physical weakness
    E. Nausea and vomiting

172. Electroencephalograms produce graphic recordings of
    A. The amount of electrical activity in a muscle or muscle group
    B. The amount of blood flow to an extremity
    C. The electrical activity of the heart
    D. The amount of electrical activity associated with brain function
    E. The level of sensory ability in a specified dermatome

173. Back and shoulder injuries due to throwing are most often caused by
    A. Improper warm-up.
    B. Poor posture.
    C. Lack of strength.
    D. Improper technique.
    E. Congenital problems.

174. Kyphosis is an abnormal curve of the spine best described as
    A. A convex curve of the upper thorax.
    B. A concave curve of the lumbar area.
    C. A lateral curve often with rotation.
    D. A concave curve of the cervical area.
    E. A lateral curve of the cervical area.

175. Why is horizontal adduction limited when an acromioclavicular separation or contusion has occurred?
    A. It forces the joint together, thus creating pressure and pain due to joint swelling.
    B. It forces the joint apart, thus stretching damaged tissue and causing pain.
    C. Horizontal adduction is not limited.
    D. It puts the rotator cuff on stretch that causes pain, thus inhibiting movement.
    E. It causes pain.

176. Which of the following is not apparent in dislocation?
    A. Loss of limb function
    B. Deformity
    C. Skin discoloration
    D. Swelling
    E. Pain

177. Arterial bleeding can usually be distinguished from venous bleeding by the characteristic of
    A. A steady flow of blood.
    B. Blood coming from the wound in spurts.
    C. A flow of dark red blood.
    D. A general ooze of blood from the tissues.
    E. Blood coming only from the wrists.

178. In nasal injuries, which of the following is absolutely contraindicated?
    A. Tilting the head back
    B. Applying gelfoam
    C. Pinching the nostrils
    D. Blowing the nose
    E. Tilting the head forward

179. Dilated and/or irregular pupils, blurring vision, and/or nystagmus are indications of
    A. Mild concussion.
    B. Unconsciousness.
    C. Brain injury.
    D. Amnesia.
    E. Myocardial ischemia.

180. A constant, involuntary movement of the eyeballs accompanying a concussion is called
    A. Anisocoria.
    B. Pupil accommodation.
    C. Nystagmus.
    D. Tinnitus.
    E. Diplopia.

181. It is often difficult to identify the time of injury to subchondral bone and articular cartilage because those structures are
    A. Not readily observable on x-ray.
    B. Insensitive (no pain receptors).
    C. Not usually a factor in activity.
    D. Seldom involved in acute trauma.
    E. Weak and are frequently injured.

182. Back pain aggravated by bending, coughing, or sneezing is a sign and symptom of previous root irritation, probably due to
    A. Disc herniation.
    B. Excessive trunk flexion.
    C. Scoliosis.
    D. Lordosis.
    E. Kyphosis.

183. The sinus tarsi is located
    A. Just posterior to the lateral malleolus.
    B. Just posterior to the medial malleolus.
    C. Just anterior to the lateral malleolus.
    D. Just anterior to the medial malleolus.
    E. Parallel to the lateral malleolus.

184. The forward subluxation of the body of one vertebra on the vertebra that is below it is called
    A. Spondylolysis.
    B. Spondylolisthesis.
    C. Sciatica.
    D. Disc herniation.
    E. Scoliosis.

185. Radicular pain refers to pain in
    A. A trigger area.
    B. The path of a peripheral nerve.
    C. Articular spaces.
    D. Acute trauma.
    E. The radius.

186. The most objective examination in evaluating nerve involvement in back trauma is a
    A. Stress test.
    B. Functional test.
    C. Reflex test.
    D. Sensory test.
    E. Neuromuscular test.

187. What does spondylolysis mean?
    A. Forward subluxation of lumbar vertebra
    B. Breaking down of a vertebral structure because of trauma or pathological defect
    C. Congenital defect or a defect caused by a disease to the vertebra—a condition that exists
    D. Any disorder of the vertebra
    E. Disc herniation

188. To what pressure point should digital pressure be applied to control bleeding from a wound in the lower leg?
    A. Brachial
    B. Femoral
    C. Subclavian
    D. Bicipital
    E. Carotid

189. Pain radiating from the low back down the buttocks to the legs can usually be related to
    A. Sciatic nerve involvement.
    B. Statis spine.
    C. Anterior compartment syndrome.
    D. Nerve root irritation.
    E. Mechanical problems.

190. Under most circumstances, brain damage will occur after _____ in the nonbreathing victim.
    A. Less than 1 minute
    B. 1–2 minutes
    C. 2–3 minutes
    D. 3–4 minutes
    E. 4–6 minutes

191. What is hyphema?
    A. A swelling or mass of blood
    B. Blood in the anterior compartment of the eye, in front of the iris
    C. Berlin's edema
    D. Blood behind the lens of the eye
    E. A pooling of blood that puts pressure on the optic nerve

192. Severe eye injury exhibits which of the following symptoms?
    A. Nausea
    B. Faintness
    C. Extreme pain
    D. Diplopia
    E. Headache

193. Entrapment of the inferior rectus muscle of the eyeball suggests
    A. Orbital rim fracture.
    B. Blow-out fracture.
    C. Glaucoma.
    D. Retinal detachment.
    E. Cataract.

194. A middle-aged woman falls unconscious in a downtown store. Her skin is cool and dry, and she is gasping. Her face is flushed, her lips are cherry red, and there is a sweet odor on her breath. What would you suspect?
    A. Cerebral hemorrhage
    B. Stroke
    C. Diabetic emergency
    D. Alcoholic stupor
    E. Carbon monoxide poisoning

195. By definition a strain is
    A. Damage to the musculotendinous unit.
    B. Damage to any soft tissue structures.
    C. Damage to the vascular structures.
    D. Damage to the ligamentous structures.
    E. Damage to the integrity of the bone.

196. Which of the following injury mechanisms would most likely produce a contusion to the eye?
    A. Being hit in the eye with a sharp object
    B. Diving too deep in the water
    C. Being hit in the eye with a racquetball ball
    D. Being hit in the face by a low flying badminton birdie
    E. Being hit in the eye with a football

197. An injury that causes blood to pool between the iris and cornea is called
    A. Ecchymosis.
    B. Hyphema.
    C. Conjunctivitis.
    D. Rebleeder.
    E. Hematoma.

198. The normal shape of the eye is like that of a basketball. If an astigmatism is present, the shape of the eye is like that of a
    A. Boomerang.
    B. Football.
    C. Bowling ball.
    D. Baseball.
    E. Frisbee®.

199. The result of a valgus force on an adolescent knee might not result in a medial collateral sprain. It could result in a/an
    A. Lateral collateral sprain.
    B. Posterior cruciate sprain.
    C. Epiphyseal fracture.
    D. Tibial tuberosity.
    E. Anterior cruciate sprain.

200. A long range of angle recession is
    A. Diabetes.
    B. Nearsightedness.
    C. Glaucoma.
    D. Farsightedness.
    E. Cataract.

201. Fractured cervical vertebrae with neurological significance are caused by
    A. Hyperextension injuries.
    B. Flexion injuries.
    C. Rotation injuries.
    D. Head-on collisions.
    E. Herniated disks.

202. Vascular injuries to the spinal cord are caused by
    A. Hyperextension injuries.
    B. Flexion injuries.
    C. Rotation injuries.
    D. Head-on collisions.
    E. Herniated disks.

203. Which carpal bone is most commonly fractured?
    A. Lunate
    B. Navicular
    C. Capitate
    D. Trapezium
    E. Pisiform

204. Neuropraxia is a concussive injury to the nerve, usually with complete recovery within
    A. 3 days.
    B. 1 week.
    C. 6 weeks.
    D. 3 months.
    E. 6 months.

205. Axonotmesis is related to trauma in which
    A. Nerve fibers are contused.
    B. Inner nerve fibers are disconnected.
    C. Outer nerve fibers are disconnected.
    D. The total nerve is disrupted.
    E. The nerve fibers are torn.

206. Neurotmesis is related to trauma in which
    A. Nerve fibers are contused.
    B. Inner nerve fibers are disconnected.
    C. Outer nerve fibers are disconnected.
    D. The total nerve is disrupted.
    E. The nerve fibers are torn.

207. Spondylosis refers to
    A. A vertebra slipping forward.
    B. A pars interarticularis defect.
    C. Degenerative changes in the spine.
    D. Ruptured disk.
    E. A congenital disorder.

208. A tooth sits in a bony cavity. The periondontal membrane surrounds it. This membrane is likened to "tiny springs" for each tooth. What is its function?
    A. It serves as a cushion and allows for better chewing ability.
    B. It serves as a cushion and protects the nerve and blood supply from impingement.
    C. It serves as a cushion and protects the bony cavity from fracture.
    D. It serves to hold the tooth firmly in the socket.
    E. It has no known value.

209. A complication of a medial ankle sprain is a/an
    A. Avulsion fracture.
    B. Strain of the peroneal tendons.
    C. Sprain of the anterior talofibular ligament
    D. Strain of the deltoid ligament.
    E. Pott's fracture.

210. An athlete has been told not to bear weight on his or her legs and has been instructed on the proper use of crutches. Which of the following statements is correct?
    A. The weight is absorbed by the athlete's axilla.
    B. The injured leg is kept in the opposite motion of the crutches.
    C. The handgrip and crutch length are adjusted so that the elbows are bent to approximately 5 degrees of flexion.
    D. The good leg leads when going up a flight of stairs.
    E. The handgrip is adjusted so that it is at the same level as the iliac crest.

211. Which of the following is not a sign or symptom of a fractured mandible?
    A. Numbness in the lower lip
    B. Malocclusion
    C. Palpable deformity at the angle
    D. With head stabilized, inability to grasp front teeth and attempt to move them
    E. Pain

212. The most commonly fractured facial bone is the
    A. Mandible.
    B. Zygomatic arch.
    C. Orbital rim of the eye.
    D. Nasal bone.
    E. Cheek bone.

213. The proximity of the fibular attachment of which of the following ligaments causes some difficulty in proper recognition?
    A. Calcaneofibular and anterior talofibular
    B. Tibiofibular and anterior talofibular
    C. Deltoid and posterior talofibular
    D. Posterior talofibular and calcaneofibular
    E. Deltoid and calcaneofibular

214. The amount of swelling in an ankle injury is indicative of the amount of
    A. Vascular damage.
    B. Structural damage.
    C. Osteochondral damage.
    D. Neuromuscular damage.
    E. Weight applied to the ankle before injury.

215. Which one of the following traumatic conditions would not show any positive radiographic findings?
    A. Osteochondral fracture
    B. Acute stress fracture
    C. Epiphyseal separation
    D. Internal derangement
    E. Orbital fracture

ANSWERS FOR SAMPLE WRITTEN QUESTIONS

DOMAIN II: RECOGNITION, EVALUATION, AND ASSESSMENT

1. C	27. C	53. A	79. B	105. A
2. B	28. B	54. C	80. B	106. C
3. A	29. B	55. D	81. B	107. A
4. B	30. C	56. D	82. C	108. B
5. B	31. D	57. D	83. B	109. B
6. A	32. D	58. B	84. D	110. C
7. C	33. A	59. B	85. B	111. E
8. C	34. C	60. D	86. B	112. D
9. D	35. A	61. B	87. A	113. C
10. A	36. B	62. C	88. C	114. B
11. D	37. C	63. A	89. D	115. D
12. C	38. D	64. B	90. A	116. B
13. B	39. D	65. B	91. C	117. D
14. B	40. B	66. E	92. B	118. A
15. E	41. C	67. B	93. E	119. A
16. D	42. C	68. D	94. B	120. D
17. C	43. C	69. E	95. D	121. C
18. A	44. A	70. A	96. C	122. C
19. C	45. D	71. A	97. B	123. B
20. C	46. D	72. D	98. D	124. C
21. B	47. C	73. A	99. B	125. B
22. A	48. A	74. A	100. D	126. A
23. D	49. A	75. C	101. C	127. B
24. A	50. D	76. B	102. E	128. E
25. B	51. E	77. B	103. C	129. D
26. A	52. A	78. C	104. C	130. B

131. C	148. A	165. B	182. A	199. C
132. D	149. A	166. C	183. C	200. C
133. C	150. C	167. B	184. B	201. B
134. C	151. B	168. C	185. B	202. A
135. A	152. B	169. A	186. C	203. B
136. D	153. B	170. C	187. B	204. C
137. E	154. D	171. D	188. B	205. C
138. E	155. A	172. D	189. A	206. D
139. A	156. B	173. D	190. E	207. C
140. C	157. E	174. A	191. B	208. B
141. C	158. C	175. A	192. C	209. A
142. A	159. A	176. C	193. A	210. D
143. A	160. D	177. B	194. C	211. D
144. B	161. B	178. D	195. A	212. D
145. D	162. B	179. C	196. C	213. D
146. A	163. A	180. C	197. B	214. A
147. D	164. C	181. B	198. B	215. D

SAMPLE WRITTEN QUESTIONS

DOMAIN III: IMMEDIATE CARE

1. When caring for a blister, you should
   A. Leave a flap of skin to protect the area after draining the blister.
   B. Puncture the blister and drain it.
   C. Remove all loose skin.
   D. Cover it with moist gauze until the blister ruptures on its own.
   E. Drain the blister and apply antibiotic ointment.

2. In treatment of a hyphema, it is recommended that the athlete
   A. Have the eye aspirated.
   B. Wear protective covering and return to competition.
   C. Take complete bed rest for 48–72 hours.
   D. Have the spine realigned by a chiropractor.
   E. Apply prescription eyedrops every 6 hours for 1 week.

3. Which method is recommended to preserve an avulsed tooth until the athlete can see a dentist?
   A. Wrap the tooth as is in moist gauze and take the tooth and athlete to the dentist.
   B. Place the tooth in a 10 percent hydrogen peroxide solution to preserve it.
   C. Scrub the tooth vigorously then place it in milk.
   D. Apply a topical dental anesthetic (Orajel®) to the tooth.
   E. Wrap the tooth in a moist hot pack.

4. When evaluating a knee injury, the athletic trainer should do all but one of the following.
   A. Observe how the athlete stands or walks.
   B. Put the athlete in a whirlpool, elevate the leg, and then palpate.
   C. Palpate.
   D. Assess for abnormal mobility.
   E. Assess function.

5. In caring for a heat-stroke victim, it is most important to
   A. Loosen the clothing and make the patient comfortable.
   B. Lower body temperature and get the patient to a hospital.
   C. Dry perspiration and have the patient drink fluids.
   D. Give fluids and have the patient take salt tablets.
   E. Replace electrolytes and remove to a sheltered environment.

6. Care for plantar warts includes
   A. Surgical removal and using doughnut padding.
   B. Removing top layers and taking an x-ray.
   C. Removing top layers and using doughnut padding.
   D. Both acid and surgical removal.
   E. Cryotherapy and removing top layers.

7. When splinting a body part, one should always
   A. Immobilize the joints above and below the fracture site.
   B. Remove all clothing from the extremity.
   C. Tighten the splint so the area becomes numb and less painful.
   D. Use a pneumatic air device.
   E. Manually test the muscle in the distal extremity.

8. Treatment of ingrown toenails should include
   A. Cutting a "V" in the nail and placing cotton under the corner of the nail.
   B. Cutting out the ingrown part of the nail and soaking the foot in Epsom salts.
   C. Shaving the top of the nail and spreading toes apart with cotton.
   D. Cleaning the dirt from the nail regularly with a nail file and soaking the nail in hot water.
   E. Surgically removing the entire toenail and allowing it to grow back properly.

9. For chemical burns of the eye, the person giving first aid should immediately
   A. Wash the eye with a solution of sodium bicarbonate.
   B. Clean the eye with a sterile cloth.
   C. Cover the eye immediately with a sterile cloth.
   D. Wash the eye with clear water.
   E. Irrigate the eye with a hypertonic glucose solution.

10. An athlete has ruptured the extensor tendon of the distal interphalangeal (DIP) joint of the ring finger. What is the recommended supportive technique during the first 4 to 6 weeks of healing?
    A. Splint the DIP joint in flexion
    B. Splint the DIP joint in extension
    C. Tape to the longest adjacent finger
    D. Tape to the most lateral finger
    E. Splint the proximal interphalangeal and DIP joints in flexion

11. Athletes who have completed the swimming leg of a triathlon go on to the biking segment. The ambient air temperature is 55°F, and the wind is steady at 15 mph. An athlete has difficulty and cannot continue riding. During your evaluation, you notice the following: the athlete is disoriented and lethargic, has garbled speech, and has a core temperature of 95°F. The athlete's respirations are shallow, and the heart rate is notably slow. The appropriate initial treatment for this athlete's condition would be to
    A. Cover the athlete with cool, damp towels and send for emergency assistance.
    B. Administer an intravenous saline solution.
    C. Move the athlete to sheltered area, wrap him or her in a warm blanket, and administer warm fluids.
    D. Transport the athlete immediately.
    E. Move the athlete to a sheltered area, administer cool fluids, and prepare the athlete for transportation.

12. Your primary concern with heat stroke is to
    A. Call the ambulance.
    B. Get fluids into the victim.
    C. Get the victim in out of the sun.
    D. Lower the victim's body temperature.
    E. Leave the patient in the same position in which he or she was found.

13. An athlete suffers a compound fracture of the middle third of the right tibia. In an initial attempt to control the bleeding, which of the following techniques would be the most effective and appropriate.
    A. Elevate the leg above the level of the heart to slow the bleeding.
    B. Gently apply sterile gauze over the wound and apply digital pressure over the femoral artery.
    C. Apply sterile gauze and direct pressure over the fracture site.
    D. Apply a tourniquet just above the knee.
    E. No action is needed because bleeding does not need to be controlled with a compound fracture.

14. The first thing you do in administering first aid to a victim with an open fracture is to
    A. Immobilize the part.
    B. Move the patient.
    C. Control hemorrhage.
    D. Apply dressing to the wound.
    E. Take vital signs.

15. A male referee running down the sidelines during a punt return suddenly grasps at his chest and collapses. His face becomes ashen and his breathing is difficult. Because you are trained in first aid, you suspect a heart attack. What would you do?
    A. Treat for shock and call for medical aid
    B. Administer fluids and apply artificial respiration
    C. Monitor the patient and send someone to activate emergency medical service
    D. Administer cardiopulmonary resuscitation
    E. Place the patient in a semireclining position and leave to get medical assistance

16. While walking in the locker room, an athlete steps on a sharp object and begins to hemorrhage from a wound in the arch of the foot. Your first response should be
    A. Application of a tourniquet.
    B. Leaving and going for medical help.
    C. Application of direct pressure.
    D. Application of digital pressure to the femoral artery.
    E. Washing the affected area.

17. In the provision of primary emergency care to an unconscious athlete with a suspected cervical spine injury, the first step is to
    A. Apply a rigid cervical collar.
    B. Place a towel in the curve of the neck.
    C. Treat the athlete for shock.
    D. Check the carotid pulse.
    E. Establish and maintain an open airway.

18. When a person is in shock, you should
    A. Administer oral fluids.
    B. Elevate the legs.
    C. Elevate the head and trunk.
    D. Induce vomiting.
    E. Assist the patient in taking his or her shock medications.

ANSWERS FOR SAMPLE WRITTEN QUESTIONS

DOMAIN III: IMMEDIATE CARE

1. C	5. B	9. D	13. B	17. E
2. C	6. C	10. B	14. C	18. B
3. A	7. A	11. C	15. C	
4. B	8. A	12. D	16. C	

SAMPLE WRITTEN QUESTIONS

DOMAIN IV: TREATMENT, REHABILITATION, AND RECONDITIONING

1. Short wave diathermy, ultrasound, and microwave diathermy as a group would be classified as
    A. Superficial heat.
    B. Deep heat.
    C. Radiant energy.
    D. Cryokinetics.
    E. Cryotherapy.

2. Which is not true about towel exercises? They
    A. Are often done for "shin splints."
    B. Require toe flexion.
    C. Require dorsiflexion.
    D. Are done for arch strains.
    E. Require abduction and adduction of the toes.

3. A metal screw or pin in the shoulder would be a contraindication for which modality?
   A. Short wave diathermy
   B. Hydrocollator packs
   C. Ultrasound
   D. Muscle stimulation
   E. Paraffin bath

4. A distance runner has developed plantar fasciitis. You would choose which of the following methods to support this injury.
   A. A medial longitudinal arch pad
   B. A lateral balance pad
   C. A heel cup
   D. An adhesive metatarsal pad
   E. A dorsal foot pad

5. A middle-aged recreational softball player comes to you complaining of low back pain secondary to increased lordosis. In general, your initial rehabilitation program should include all of the following except
   A. Bent-knee sit-ups.
   B. Proprioceptive neuromuscular facilitation hamstring stretching.
   C. Resistive hamstring curls.
   D. William's flexion exercises.
   E. Moist-heat application.

6. Active assistive exercises are given when
   A. Resistance can be given through a partial range of motion.
   B. Maximum resistance through the full range of motion can be given.
   C. Minimum resistance through the full range of motion can be given.
   D. Fifty percent of the range of motion is restored, compared with the uninvolved side.
   E. The strength of muscles is not sufficient to perform the fullest range of motion possible.

7. One megahertz is the wavelength of which modality?
   A. Short wave diathermy
   B. Electrical stimulation
   C. Microwave diathermy
   D. Ultrasound
   E. Ultrawave diathermy

8. Which of the following modalities uses 27 MHz as its wavelength?
   A. Short wave diathermy
   B. Long wave diathermy
   C. Microwave diathermy
   D. Ultrasound
   E. Ultrawave diathermy

9. Active internal rotation of the glenohumeral joint is controlled primarily by which one of the following muscles?
   A. Coracobrachial
   B. Smaller pectoral
   C. Infraspinous
   D. Deltoid
   E. Subscapular

10. Agitation of the water by introduction of air into the whirlpool bath has the effect of
    A. Providing a gentle massage to the part that is being treated.
    B. Increasing the joint motion of the extremity that is being treated.
    C. Mechanically dilating the arteries.
    D. Reducing pressure on the injured part.
    E. Raising the body temperature considerably.

11. An athlete returns from the physician with a prescription that reads "ice baths PRN." The athlete should be given an ice bath
    A. Before 12:00 noon.
    B. After each running session.
    C. Before going to bed.
    D. Before each running session.
    E. As needed by the athlete.

12. During diathermy application, electromagnetic energy is used to heat the deeper tissues by a method of heat production called
    A. Radiation.
    B. Modulation.
    C. Conversion.
    D. Convection.
    E. Conduction.

13. During the healing process following an injury, which of the following activities occurs initially?
    A. Collagen fibers are realigned according to tensile forces.

B. Fibroblasts lay down collagen fibers.

C. Scar tissue is completely reabsorbed because of the increased vascularization.

D. Leukocytes and phagocytes collect in the injured area.

E. Fibroblastic proliferation leads to increased production of histamine, which decreases blood flow.

14. During the rehabilitation of Osgood-Schlatter disease, which of the following exercises should be avoided?
    A. Seated lateral pulls
    B. Seated rowing
    C. Bench press
    D. Quadriceps setting exercises
    E. Quadriceps plyometrics

15. Electrical stimulation applied with a short phase duration at an intensity that does not cause a muscle contraction is thought to control pain through
    A. The pattern theory.
    B. Enkephalin release.
    C. The gate-control theory.
    D. The specificity theory.
    E. The central biasing mechanism.

16. Following a severe injury, the athlete typically experiences a "grieving response." Research has shown that the typical sequence of this response is
    A. Depression, denial, anger, and acceptance.
    B. Denial, depression, anger, and acceptance.
    C. Anger, depression, denial, and acceptance.
    D. Denial, anger, depression, and acceptance.
    E. Depression, anger, denial, and acceptance.

17. Pigmentation is an aspect of which modality?
    A. Ultraviolet
    B. Infrared
    C. Vapocoolants
    D. Hyperbaric chamber
    E. Paraffin

18. After major knee surgery with complications and 15 days of complete bed rest, you are instructed by the physician to implement a one-legged, nonaffected bicycle ergometer program as a part of the rehabilitation program. As a result of this program, you would expect the athlete to have increases in all of these cardiovascular areas **except**
    A. Vo_2max
    B. Cardiac output
    C. Resting heart rate
    D. Arteriovenous oxygen difference
    E. Stroke volume

19. Heat causes resting capillaries to dilate and thus provides the physiological benefits of
    A. Decreasing antibodies and slowing the metabolic process.
    B. Increasing antibodies and diminishing the metabolic process.
    C. Increasing antibodies and increasing the metabolic process.
    D. Decreasing antibodies and increasing the metabolic process.
    E. Decreasing antibodies and maintaining the metabolic process at its pretreatment level.

20. Massage is contraindicated in the presence of
    A. Acute inflammatory process.
    B. Joint contracture.
    C. Scar tissue.
    D. Muscle spasm.
    E. Edema.

21. According to most authorities, one of the most important objectives in conditioning is
    A. Warm-up.
    B. Flexibility.
    C. Running.
    D. Endurance.
    E. Momentum.

22. The "static hang" is an exercise for
    A. Shoulder dislocation.
    B. Elbow.
    C. Back.
    D. Torso.
    E. Legs.

23. Increased chronaxy is a physiological effect of
    A. Cold.
    B. Heat.
    C. Ultrasound.
    D. Ultraviolet.
    E. Radiant energy.

24. The initial phase of a rehabilitation program is focused on
    A. Tissue healing.
    B. Restoring passive range of motion.
    C. Restoring active range of motion.
    D. Facilitating muscular strength.
    E. Restoring proprioceptive function.

25. The primary benefit of cold application during the immediate treatment of an injury is that it
    A. Decreases the amount of swelling.
    B. Decreases the cell's metabolic need for oxygen.
    C. Decreases the viscosity of fluids in the injured area.
    D. Decreases the amount of hemorrhage that occurs.
    E. Increases the amount of plasma proteins escaping into the surrounding tissues.

26. The primary principle in the treatment of muscular weakness is
    A. Increased range of motion.
    B. Synergetic actions of the muscle.
    C. Bilateral activity.
    D. Graded resistance.
    E. Tonic contractures.

27. Proprioceptive exercises such as using the balance board increase the athlete's _____ awareness of lower-extremity structures.
    A. Metabolic
    B. Ergonomic
    C. Visual
    D. Cognitive
    E. Kinesthetic

28. To know that a muscle truly has strength corresponding to the amount of weight lifted, the supervisor should rule out or prevent
    A. Momentum.
    B. Astigmatism.
    C. Chondromalacia.

    D. Isolated work.
    E. Velocity.

29. The use of electricity to introduce ions into the tissues is
    A. Phonophoresis.
    B. Interferential stimulation.
    C. Iontophoresis.
    D. Galvanic stimulation.
    E. Dermophoresis.

30. Transcutaneous electrical nerve stimulation (TENS) is an acceptable modality for use in
    A. Pain management.
    B. Increasing the healing rate.
    C. Combating inflammation.
    D. Decreasing effusion.
    E. Increasing range of motion.

31. After using the whirlpool for a subacute injury in the lower extremity, the patient should
    A. Elevate his or her leg.
    B. Stand in ice water.
    C. Turn off the turbine.
    D. Exercise his or her leg.
    E. Wrap his or her leg in an elastic bandage.

32. Contraindications for using **short wave diathermy** include
    A. Metal implants, sensory loss, and hemorrhage.
    B. Metal implants, chronic inflammation, and hemorrhage.
    C. Chronic inflammation, sensory loss, and hemorrhage.
    D. Metal implants, sensory loss, and chronic inflammation.
    E. Chronic inflammation, metal implants, and pain.

33. Massage helps increase circulation and also helps in
    A. Decreasing lymphatic and venous circulation.
    B. Eliminating toxins.
    C. Slowing cellular metabolism.
    D. Increasing scar formation.
    E. Decreasing blood flow to major organs.

34. Cryokinetics is the use of cold to
    A. Induce motion.
    B. Control symptoms while initiating exercise.
    C. Enhance the healing rate.
    D. Increase blood flow.
    E. Decrease inflammation.

35. Mottling is a/an
    A. Pathological development related to excessive deep heat.
    B. Spotty reddening caused by excessive histamine release because of heat exposure.
    C. Patchy blue color caused by lack of oxygen to the tissues.
    D. Histamine reaction that leads to hemorrhage.
    E. Adverse reaction to contrast bath.

36. Ice used in cryokinetics should usually be used for
    A. 5–10 minutes.
    B. 15–20 minutes.
    C. 20–30 minutes.
    D. 30–60 minutes.
    E. 60–75 minutes.

37. The therapeutic tool that is most beneficial in athletes because it best represents the functional activity of athletics is
    A. Exercise.
    B. Cryotherapy.
    C. Electrical stimulation.
    D. Whirlpool.
    E. Contrast bath.

38. The loss of vascular integrity is the only proven indication for what modality?
    A. Paraffin bath
    B. Cryotherapy
    C. Microwave diathermy
    D. Contrast bath
    E. Electrical stimulation

39. Loss of vascular integrity is an indication for
    A. Electrical stimulation.
    B. Ultrasound.
    C. Short wave diathermy.
    D. Contrast.
    E. Whirlpool.

40. Which of the following is not an acceptable method of I.C.E.?
    A. Ice bag held on with a compression wrap and injured part elevated
    B. Injured part elevated with wet compression wrap and ice
    C. Compression wrap in a slush bath
    D. Elevation with an ice bag and pneumatic splint
    E. Slush bucket

41. Hemorrhage control is an indication for
    A. Cryotherapy.
    B. Thermotherapy.
    C. Whirlpool.
    D. Electrical stimulation.
    E. Ultrasound.

42. When treating an appendage, the water temperature for a hot whirlpool should be
    A. 86°F–92°F.
    B. 94°F–100°F.
    C. 102°F–110°F.
    D. 110°F–120°F.
    E. 115°F–120°F.

43. The inverse square law states that
    A. The farther away the source, the greater the intensity in linear proportions.
    B. The closer the source, the greater the intensity in linear proportions.
    C. The farther away the source, the less the intensity in a squared relationship.
    D. The closer the source, the less the intensity in a squared relationship.
    E. The farther away the source, the greater the intensity in a squared relationship.

44. An induction coil places the patient
    A. As a part of the circuit.
    B. Under an A, B, C, or D director.
    C. In an electromagnetic field.
    D. In position of high impedance.
    E. In position of low impedance.

45. A chronaxy value refers to
    A. Cholinesterase level.
    B. Nerve conduction velocity.
    C. Level necrosis development.
    D. Nerve excitation level.
    E. Action potential.

46. To be lethal to microorganisms, the bactericidal effect of ultraviolet light requires an intensity of
    A. Several times less than the minimal effective dose.
    B. At least an MED dose.
    C. Twice as much as a minimal effective dose.
    D. Four times the minimal effective dose.
    E. A variable minimal effective dose.

47. All agents used in the treatment of injuries are called
    A. Antibiotics.
    B. Therapeutic exercises.
    C. Rehabilitation apparatus.
    D. Therapeutic modalities.
    E. Analgesics.

48. Which is **not** a consideration regarding the use of heat?
    A. Never apply heat where sensation is intact.
    B. Never apply heat immediately after an injury.
    C. Never apply heat where there is decreased arterial circulation.
    D. Never apply heat directly over the genital area.
    E. Never apply heat where there is a loss of sensation.

49. Ice, compression, and elevation do not assist with
    A. Lowering metabolism.
    B. Creating pressure.
    C. Equalizing pressure.
    D. Lowering hydrostatic pressure.
    E. Increasing basal metabolic rate.

50. Metal implants are a contraindication of which modality?
    A. Electrical stimulation
    B. Traction
    C. Short wave diathermy
    D. Contrast
    E. Whirlpool

51. Which of the following is not a contraindication for transcutaneous electrical nerve stimulation (TENS)?
    A. Patients with cardiac pacemaker
    B. Over carotid sinus
    C. Pregnancy

D. Over lumbar spine
E. Over laryngeal and pharyngeal muscles

52. Which of the following is not an electrical stimulation point?
    A. Acupuncture points.
    B. Motor point.
    C. Trigger point.
    D. Beta point.
    E. Dermatome.

53. Deep-heating modalities have increased the temperature of deep tissue by
    A. 3°F–5°F.
    B. 7°F–9°F.
    C. 11°F–13°F.
    D. 15°F–17°F.
    E. 18°F–20°F.

54. What is the frequency of the sound waves used in therapeutic ultrasound?
    A. 1 Mc
    B. 10 Mc
    C. 100 Mc
    D. 1000 Mc
    E. 1,000,000 Mc

55. What causes the ultrasound transducer crystal to vibrate and create sound waves?
    A. It is mechanically shaken.
    B. It is chemically stimulated.
    C. It is sensitive to electrical polarity.
    D. It is sensitive to a patient's electrical potential.
    E. It has reached chronaxy.

56. The whirlpool is used to achieve localized superficial heat and
    A. Pulse stability.
    B. Vascular exercise.
    C. Increased cellular permeability.
    D. Increased range of motion.
    E. Decrease inflammation.

57. One goal or principle of therapeutic exercise is to restore
    A. Full range of motion.
    B. Anabolic support program.
    C. Strength before flexibility.
    D. Flexibility before strength.
    E. Anaerobic before aerobic.

58. Short wave diathermy can increase the temperature to deep tissues by
    A. 1°F–3°F.
    B. 3°F–5°F.
    C. 5°F–7°F.
    D. 7°F–9°F.
    E. 10°F–12°F.

59. _____ is given to constrict superficial blood vessels, thus producing ideal inhibition of circulation:
    A. Enzyme therapy
    B. Cryotherapy
    C. Ultrasonics
    D. Thermotherapy
    E. Electrotherapy

60. Superficial heat causes
    A. A faster chemical reaction.
    B. A slower chemical reaction.
    C. An increased reaction time.
    D. A slower reaction time.
    E. Decreased polarity.

61. Superficial heat will
    A. Aid membrane permeability.
    B. Increase membrane permeability.
    C. Increase membrane permeability greatly.
    D. Stop membrane attempts for permeability.
    E. Not affect permeability.

62. Superficial is considered heat to the depth of
    A. 3–5 mm.
    B. 7–9 mm.
    C. 1 inch.
    D. 2 inches.
    E. 3–5 inches.

63. What is the depth penetration of heat obtained from whirlpools and hot packs?
    A. 3–5 inches
    B. 1 mm
    C. 2–4 cm
    D. 3–5 mm
    E. 1–2 inches

64. Corresponding with an increase in strength, one should increase or at least maintain
    A. Agility.
    B. Mobility.
    C. Flexibility
    D. Cardiovascular fitness.
    E. Endurance.

65. In treatments with ultrasonic energy, a coupling medium is used because ultrasonic energy
    A. Cannot be transmitted through the air.
    B. Reduces the athlete's sensitivity to the passage of energy.
    C. Reduces the force of the vibrations of energy.
    D. Diminishes the hazard of deep-tissue damage.
    E. Minimizes deflection of the energy by the skin.

66. Manual muscle testing does not attempt to precisely quantify the amount of force generated by a muscle group. A major purpose of manual muscle testing is to
    A. Compare the injured limb's range of motion with the opposing extremity.
    B. Objectively measure the muscle function of the injured limb.
    C. Rehabilitate the muscles of the injured limb.
    D. Reeducate the neurological functions of the injured limb.
    E. Compare the injured limb's muscle function with that of the opposing extremity.

67. The most important area to gain flexibility in knee rehabilitation involves the
    A. Hamstring muscles.
    B. Quadriceps muscles.
    C. Gluteal muscles.
    D. Gastrocnemius muscles.
    E. Ligaments.

68. For contact sports, it is generally considered necessary to develop quadriceps muscle strength to at least
    A. One half of body weight.
    B. One third of body weight.
    C. One fourth of body weight.
    D. One fifth of body weight.
    E. Three fourths of body weight.

69. Which is not a type of massage?
    A. Pétrissage
    B. Effleurage
    C. Compressing
    D. Tapotement
    E. Vibration

70. The Food and Drug Administration (FDA) requires hospitals to have a _____ and a _____ check every _____ on all therapeutic modalities.
    A. Calibration, safety, 6 months
    B. Power, electrical, year
    C. Computerized, unit, 3 months
    D. Power, safety, 2 years
    E. Safety, electrical, year

71. Conduction may be defined as
    A. Changing one form of energy to a heat form.
    B. Heat transfer by air currents.
    C. Energy transfer from a hot body to a cooler body through distance in a gas medium.
    D. Heat transfer by direct contact.
    E. The removal of thermal energy by changing a liquid to a gas.

72. Radiation may be defined as
    A. Changing one form of energy to a heat form.
    B. Heat transfer by air currents.
    C. Energy transfer from a hot body to a cooler body through distance in a gas medium.
    D. Heat transfer by direct contact.
    E. The removal of thermal energy by changing a liquid to a gas.

73. Athletes should treat themselves
    A. Only when properly trained.
    B. Only when supervised.
    C. Only after procedure becomes routine.
    D. Never.
    E. Only when injured.

74. Infrared and ultraviolet radiation would be classified as
    A. Pharmacotherapeutic.
    B. Deep heating.
    C. Radiant energy.
    D. Cryokinetics.
    E. Cryotherapy.

75. Warm whirlpool and paraffin baths could be classified as
    A. Cryokinetics.
    B. Cryotherapy.
    C. Mechanical traction.
    D. Moist heat.
    E. Deep heat.

76. Palmar and dorsal interosseous muscles of the hand primarily control which of the following movements of the digits?
    A. Abduction/adduction
    B. Abduction/flexion
    C. Adduction/flexion
    D. Abduction/extension
    E. Adduction/extension

77. The inflammatory mediator that functions to inhibit blood clotting is
    A. Prostaglandins.
    B. Heparin.
    C. Histamine.
    D. Thrombin.
    E. Leukotrienes.

78. As a group, ice massage and exercise, slush bath and range of motion, ice pack and gait practice would be classified as
    A. Superficial heat.
    B. Deep heat.
    C. Radiant energy.
    D. Cryokinetics.
    E. Cryotherapy.

79. Decreased fluid viscosity is a physiological effect of
    A. Cold.
    B. Heat.
    C. Ultrasound.
    D. Ultraviolet.
    E. Radiant energy.

80. Decreased cell permeability is a physiological effect of
    A. Cold.
    B. Heat.
    C. Ultrasound.
    D. Ultraviolet.
    E. Radiant energy.

81. Increased histamine production is a physiological effect of
    A. Cold.
    B. Heat.
    C. Ultrasound.
    D. Ultraviolet.
    E. Radiant energy.

82. Cavitation is a physiological effect of
    A. Cold.
    B. Heat.
    C. Ultrasound.
    D. Ultraviolet.
    E. Radiant energy.

83. Proper hamstring strength is generally considered to be about
    A. Three fourths of quadriceps strength or better.
    B. One half to three fourths of quadriceps strength.
    C. One third to one half of quadriceps strength.
    D. One fourth to one third of quadriceps strength.
    E. One fourth to one half of quadriceps strength.

84. Therapeutic exercise must involve which of the following principles to functionally protect a joint with strength during competition?
    A. Full range of motion and the overload principle
    B. Full range of motion and static stretching
    C. Static stretching and high repetitions
    D. High repetition and Demeter's principle
    E. High repetition and the overload principle

85. A principle to follow in flexibility exercises after injury is
    A. Ballistic stretching.
    B. Overload principle.
    C. Demeter's principle.
    D. Isolate the area.
    E. Daily adjusted progressive resistive exercise (DAPRE).

86. Increased chemical activity is a physiological effect of
    A. Cold.
    B. Heat.
    C. Ultrasound.
    D. Ultraviolet.
    E. Radiant energy.

87. Exercises to protect the shoulder from anterior dislocation include
    A. Circumduction and flexion.
    B. Flexion and extension.
    C. Abduction and external rotation.
    D. Adduction and internal rotation.
    E. Abduction and internal rotation.

88. Because the elbow tends to lose range of motion (ROM) with forced stretching, it is recommended that elbow ROM be rehabilitated by
    A. Passive exercise.
    B. Active exercise.
    C. Manipulative exercise.
    D. Isometric exercise.
    E. Strength training.

89. Acute trauma is an indication for
    A. Cryotherapy.
    B. Thermotherapy.
    C. Whirlpool.
    D. Electrical stimulation.
    E. Ultrasound.

90. When rehabilitating an athlete who is suffering from a laterally subluxing patella secondary to an increased Q angle, which muscle should be emphasized?
    A. Tensor muscle of the fascia lata
    B. Gracilis muscle
    C. Rectus muscle of the thigh
    D. Pes anserine
    E. Oblique medial vastus muscle

91. Increased oxygen and carbon dioxide tension are physiological effects of
    A. Cold.
    B. Heat.
    C. Ultrasound.
    D. Ultraviolet.
    E. Radiant energy.

92. Which is not a therapeutic exercise principle pertaining to strength?
    A. Pain free
    B. No ballistic motion
    C. No momentum
    D. Overload
    E. Gradualism

93. Débridement is an indication for
    A. Cryotherapy.
    B. Thermotherapy.
    C. Whirlpool.
    D. Electrical stimulation.
    E. Ultrasound.

94. Therapeutic exercise involving any joint must ensure
    A. Proper balance of strength to all concerned muscles.
    B. Proper ligamentous integrity.
    C. At least double strength.
    D. Shortening of the musculature.
    E. Lengthening of the musculature.

95. The most important areas to strengthen in knee rehabilitation involve the
    A. Quadriceps and hamstring muscles.
    B. Gluteal and quadriceps muscles.
    C. Quadriceps and gastrocnemius muscles.
    D. Gluteal and hamstring muscles.
    E. Gluteal and gastrocnemius muscles.

96. Massage and traction as a group would be classified as
    A. Cryokinetics.
    B. Cryotherapy.
    C. Mechanical agents.
    D. Moist heat.
    E. Radiant energy.

97. Electrode placement for transcutaneous electrical nerve stimulation (TENS) would not be considered at which of the following points?
    A. Location of greatest tenderness
    B. Pedal pressure points
    C. Specific dermatomes or spinal segments
    D. Superficial points along peripheral nerves
    E. Contiguous to the painful site

98. Deep heat can heat tissues as deep as
    A. 3–5 mm.
    B. 10 mm.
    C. 1 inch.
    D. 2 inches.
    E. 3 inches.

99. Phlebitis is a contraindication for which modality?
    A. Cryotherapy
    B. Thermotherapy
    C. Whirlpool
    D. Electrical stimulation
    E. Ultrasound

100. Peripheral vascular disease is a contraindication to which modality?
    A. Cryotherapy
    B. Thermotherapy
    C. Whirlpool
    D. Electrical stimulation
    E. Ultrasound

101. Which modality is contraindicated before muscular activity?
    A. Cryotherapy
    B. Thermotherapy
    C. Whirlpool
    D. Electrical stimulation
    E. Ultrasound

102. Which modality is contraindicated in conditions with unmyelinated nerve?
    A. Cryotherapy
    B. Thermotherapy
    C. Whirlpool
    D. Electrical stimulation
    E. Ultrasound

103. Infrared radiation, a hydrocollator, and a whirlpool as a group would be classified as
    A. Superficial heat.
    B. Deep heat.
    C. Radiant energy.
    D. Cryokinetics.
    E. Cryotherapy.

104. Skin infections are a contraindication to which modality?
    A. Cryotherapy
    B. Thermotherapy
    C. Whirlpool
    D. Electrical stimulation
    E. Ultrasound

105. Malignancy is a contraindication to which modality?
    A. Cryotherapy
    B. Thermotherapy
    C. Whirlpool
    D. Electrical stimulation
    E. Ultrasound

106. Internal compression is best obtained by
   A. Ice.
   B. Cryo cuff.
   C. Elevation.
   D. Elastic bandages.
   E. Muscular contraction.

107. Thermotherapy treatments are usually not productive if their frequency is less than
   A. Weekly.
   B. Three times a week.
   C. Daily.
   D. Three times a day.
   E. Once a month.

108. Endurance is a factor to be considered in therapeutic exercise. The two most important factors are
   A. Agility and strength.
   B. Strength and bulk.
   C. Flexibility and strength.
   D. Girth and strength.
   E. Agility and girth.

109. The initial reaction to local intense heat is
   A. Vasodilation.
   B. Vasoconstriction.
   C. Histamine release.
   D. Sedative in nature.
   E. Pain.

110. The initial reaction to local intense cold is
   A. Vasodilation.
   B. Vasoconstriction.
   C. Withdrawal.
   D. Pain.
   E. Histamine release.

111. Which would be best to increase range of motion after cast removal?
   A. Cold
   B. Infrared
   C. Paraffin bath
   D. Whirlpool
   E. Hydrocollator pack

112. Which would be best to decrease distal extremity arthritic pain?
   A. Cold whirlpool
   B. Infrared
   C. Paraffin bath
   D. Vapocoolant spray
   E. Hydrocollator pack

113. Which would be best to decrease acute inflammation?
   A. Cold
   B. Infrared
   C. Paraffin bath
   D. Whirlpool
   E. Hydrocollator pack

114. Which would be best to treat conjunctivitis and sinusitis?
   A. Cold
   B. Infrared
   C. Paraffin bath
   D. Whirlpool
   E. Hydrocollator pack

115. Which would be best to treat spasticity?
   A. Cold
   B. Infrared
   C. Paraffin bath
   D. Whirlpool
   E. Hydrocollator pack

116. In which order do sensations to cold happen?
   A. Cold, burning, aching, numbing
   B. Cold, aching, burning, numbing
   C. Cold, numbing, burning, aching
   D. Numbing, burning, aching, cold
   E. Cold, burning, numbing, aching

117. How far away from the treated area should a vapocoolant spray, such as ethyl chloride, be used?
   A. 6–12 inches
   B. 12–16 inches
   C. 18–36 inches
   D. 36–48 inches
   E. 48–60 inches

118. How fast should an athletic trainer move a vapocoolant spray, such as fluoromethane, when treating the affected area?
   A. 1 inch/s
   B. 4 inches/s
   C. 6 inches/s
   D. 8 inches/s
   E. 12 inches/s

119. What therapeutic qualities are included in ultrasound?
    A. Thermal and mechanical
    B. Light and electrical
    C. Thermal and chemical
    D. Chemical and mechanical
    E. Light and mechanical

120. What order of exercises can most safely be used in cryokinetics?
    A. Passive range of motion (ROM), active ROM, resistive ROM, weight-bearing activity.
    B. Weigh-bearing activity, passive ROM, active ROM, resistive ROM.
    C. Passive ROM, resistive ROM, weight-bearing activity, active ROM.
    D. Active ROM, resistive ROM, weight-bearing activity, passive ROM.
    E. Active ROM, weight-bearing activity, resistive ROM, passive ROM.

121. Hydrating the area is an effect of
    A. Whirlpool.
    B. Elevation.
    C. Massage.
    D. Compression wrap.
    E. Ultrasound.

122. Flexibility exercises require static stretching to
    A. Actually elongate tissue and prevent damage.
    B. Create proper blood flow.
    C. Encourage position sense.
    D. Make rapid flexibility progress.
    E. Decrease pain during exercise.

123. Proper heat intensity is at a level that
    A. Creates mottling.
    B. Feels hot but is not quite strong enough to mottle the skin.
    C. Is comfortably warm.
    D. Varies with the type of pathology.
    E. Varies with the type of heat source applied.

124. Generally the optimum duration for thermotherapy is
    A. 10 minutes.
    B. 20 minutes.
    C. 30 minutes.
    D. 40 minutes.
    E. 60 minutes.

125. Which of the Williams' flexion exercises stretches the opposite of a hip flexor?
    A. Pelvic tilt
    B. Curl up
    C. Both knees to chest
    D. Alternate knee to chest
    E. Both legs straight up

126. Slush bath, ice massage, ethyl chloride, and an ice bag as a group would be classified as
    A. Superficial heat.
    B. Deep heat.
    C. Radiant energy.
    D. Cryokinetics.
    E. Cryotherapy.

127. After a knee injury and before competition, an athlete should condition the injured area to have proper
    A. Strength, range of motion, and flexibility.
    B. Strength, flexibility, and stability.
    C. Range of motion, girth, and stability.
    D. Girth, flexibility, and agility.
    E. Range of motion, strength, and stability.

128. The cosine law states that
    A. As the angle of incidence decreases from 90 degrees, the intensity decreases.
    B. Intensity is greatest at an angle of incidence of 180 degrees.
    C. As the angle of incidence decreases from 90 degrees the intensity increases.
    D. Radiation angulation has no relationship to intensity.
    E. As the angle of incidence increases from 180 degrees, the intensity increases.

129. A hydrocollator unit stores water for use at what temperature?
    A. 102°F–110°F
    B. 120°F–130°F
    C. 150°F–195°F
    D. 200°F–210°F
    E. 215°F–225°F

130. For which modality is 118°F–126°F the proper temperature?
    A. Whirlpool
    B. Paraffin bath
    C. Hydrocollator packs
    D. Ultrasound
    E. Cryotherapy

131. In the case of injury to the lateral ankle ligaments, the strength of which muscles should be emphasized to compensate for any residual laxity?
    A. Anterior tibial, posterior tibial
    B. Anterior tibial, long flexor of the great toe
    C. Gastrocnemius, posterior tibial
    D. Long peroneal, short peroneal
    E. Long flexor of the great toe, posterior tibial, long flexor of the toes

132. To ensure their safe operation, whirlpool motors must be connected to
    A. A circuit breaker.
    B. A ground fault interrupter.
    C. A hospital-grade plug.
    D. A fast-blow fuse.
    E. A dedicated circuit.

133. Which of the following should be avoided during the initial stages of a treatment or rehabilitation program of a subluxing glenohumeral joint?
    A. Controlling pain through electrical stimulation
    B. Isometric muscle strengthening exercises
    C. Passive range of motion exercises
    D. Joint mobilization
    E. Gentle stretching

134. The stretch reflex relates to
    A. Strength principles of therapeutic exercise.
    B. Gradualism.
    C. Flexibility principles of therapeutic exercises.
    D. DeLorme's theory.
    E. DAPRE.

135. Short wave diathermy condenser plates place the patient
    A. As a part of the circuit.
    B. Under an A, B, C, or D director.
    C. In an electromagnetic field.
    D. In a position of high impedance.
    E. At greater risk for refraction.

136. Which of the following modalities uses 2450 MHz as its wavelength?
    A. Short wave diathermy
    B. Long wave diathermy
    C. Microwave diathermy
    D. Ultrasound
    E. Ultrawave diathermy

137. Flexion and extension of the glenohumeral joint occur in the _____ plane around a _____ axis.
    A. Frontal, anterior/posterior
    B. Transverse, longitudinal
    C. Frontal, coronal
    D. Sagittal, coronal
    E. Transverse, longitudinal

138. In the seated position, the amount of dorsiflexion of the ankle should be approximately
    A. 30 degrees.
    B. 40 degrees.
    C. 50 degrees.
    D. 60 degrees.
    E. 70 degrees.

139. Contrast bath is used to get optimum
    A. Temperature change.
    B. Vascular exercise.
    C. Cellular permeability.
    D. Metabolic rate.
    E. Healing rate.

140. How high can ultrasound increase the internal temperature of tissues?
    A. 1°F–3°F
    B. 3°F–5°F
    C. 5°F–7°F
    D. 7°F–9°F
    E. 10°F–12°F

141. Which of the following modalities uses frequencies above 17,000 cycles/s?
    A. High voltage pulsed stimulation
    B. Low voltage galvanic
    C. Short wave diathermy
    D. Microwave diathermy
    E. Ultrasound

142. Which of the following modalities uses beamed electromagnetic energy?
    A. Faradic electrical stimulation
    B. High voltage pulsed stimulation
    C. Low voltage galvanic
    D. Short wave diathermy
    E. Microwave diathermy

143. Which of the following modalities consists of two circuits?
    A. Faradic electrical stimulation
    B. High voltage pulsed stimulation
    C. Low voltage galvanic
    D. Short wave diathermy
    E. Microwave diathermy

144. Which modality is involved when high frequencies are reflected from dense biologic interfaces?
    A. High voltage pulsed stimulation
    B. Low voltage galvanic
    C. Short wave diathermy
    D. Microwave diathermy
    E. Ultrasound

145. A piezoelectric crystal is employed in which modality?
    A. High voltage pulsed stimulation
    B. Low voltage galvanic
    C. Short wave diathermy
    D. Microwave diathermy
    E. Ultrasound

146. Using two active electrodes and one dispersive electrode is a technique in which modality?
    A. Faradic electrical stimulation
    B. High voltage pulsed stimulation
    C. Low voltage galvanic stimulation
    D. Microwave diathermy
    E. Ultrasound

147. A therapeutic intensity range between 0.5 and 2.0 W/cm² is usually related to which modality?
    A. High voltage pulsed stimulation
    B. Low voltage galvanic
    C. Microwave diathermy
    D. Short wave diathermy
    E. Ultrasound

148. Which of the following modalities stimulates denervated muscle?
    A. Faradic electrical stimulation
    B. High voltage pulsed stimulation
    C. Low voltage galvanic
    D. Short wave diathermy
    E. Microwave diathermy

149. Sinusoidal waves relate to which modality?
    A. Faradic electrical stimulation
    B. Long wave diathermy
    C. Ultrasound
    D. Microwave diathermy
    E. Low voltage galvanic

150. You would need to consider the buildup of acoustical impedance with which modality?
    A. Microwave diathermy
    B. Ultrasound
    C. Long wave diathermy
    D. Short wave diathermy
    E. Faradic electrical stimulation

151. A rheobase value refers to
    A. Cholinesterase level.
    B. Nerve conduction velocity.
    C. Level of necrosis development.
    D. Nerve excitation level.
    E. Action potential.

152. Convection may be defined as
    A. Changing one form of energy to a heat form.
    B. Heat transfer by air currents.
    C. Energy transfer from a hot body to a cooler body through distance in a gas medium.
    D. Heat transfer by direct contact.
    E. The removal of thermal energy by changing a liquid to a gas.

153. Conversion may be defined as
    A. Changing one form of energy to a heat form.
    B. Heat transfer by air currents.
    C. Energy transfer from a hot body to a cooler body through distance in a gas medium.
    D. Heat transfer by direct contact.
    E. The removal of thermal energy by changing a liquid to a gas.

154. Which modality causes ion movement?
    A. Faradic
    B. High voltage pulsed stimulation
    C. Low voltage galvanic
    D. Russian
    E. Interferential

155. Which modality is used for iontophoresis?
    A. Faradic
    B. High voltage pulsed stimulation
    C. Low voltage galvanic
    D. Russian
    E. Interferential

156. Which modality is most indicated in low back strains with no additional complications?
    A. Traction
    B. Ultrasound
    C. Massage
    D. Vapocoolants
    E. Iontophoresis

157. Which modality is used to mechanically remove edema?
    A. Traction
    B. Ultrasound
    C. Nonsteroidal anti-inflammatory drugs (NSAIDs)
    D. Vapocoolants
    E. Iontophoresis

158. Which modality is used to relieve nerve root compression?
    A. Traction
    B. Ultrasound
    C. Massage
    D. Vapocoolants
    E. Iontophoresis

159. Which modality is used to stretch adhesions?
    A. Traction
    B. Ultrasound
    C. Massage
    D. Vapocoolants
    E. Iontophoresis

160. Stroking is a part of which form of massage?
    A. Tapotement
    B. Effleurage
    C. Pétrissage
    D. Friction
    E. Vibration

161. Kneading is a part of which form of massage?
    A. Tapotement
    B. Effleurage
    C. Pétrissage
    D. Friction
    E. Vibration

162. Pounding is a part of which form of massage?
    A. Tapotement
    B. Effleurage
    C. Pétrissage
    D. Friction
    E. Vibration

163. Rubbing with fingers and thumb is a part of which form of massage?
    A. Tapotement
    B. Effleurage
    C. Pétrissage
    D. Friction
    E. Vibration

164. Which form of massage produces a beat?
    A. Tapotement
    B. Effleurage
    C. Pétrissage
    D. Friction
    E. Vibration

165. Which form of massage uses a gentle milking action?
    A. Tapotement
    B. Effleurage
    C. Pétrissage
    D. Friction
    E. Vibration

166. Which form of massage stretches adhesions?
    A. Tapotement
    B. Effleurage
    C. Pétrissage
    D. Friction
    E. Vibration

167. Which form of massage is used over scar tissue?
    A. Tapotement
    B. Effleurage
    C. Pétrissage
    D. Friction
    E. Vibration

168. Because pain is useful to guard against overstress, transcutaneous electrical nerve stimulation (TENS) should not be used
    A. Before stressful physical activity.
    B. During stressful physical activity.
    C. After stressful physical activity.
    D. With ice after a stressful activity.
    E. With heat before a stressful activity.

169. The angle of pull in cervical traction should be
    A. 15 degrees.
    B. 25 degrees.
    C. 30 degrees.
    D. 45 degrees.
    E. 60 degrees.

170. Cervical traction should pull the neck into
     A. Flexion.
     B. Extension.
     C. Abduction.
     D. Hyperextension.
     E. Adduction

171. The use of goggles is required with which modality?
     A. Ultraviolet
     B. Infrared
     C. Vapocoolants
     D. Hyperbaric
     E. Paraffin

172. Which modality provides the most superficial heat?
     A. Ultraviolet
     B. Infrared
     C. Vapocoolants
     D. Hyperbaric
     E. Paraffin

173. Vitamin D activation is an aspect of which modality?
     A. Ultraviolet
     B. Infrared
     C. Vapocoolants
     D. Hyperbaric
     E. Paraffin

174. Which exercise is not considered a Williams' flexion exercise?
     A. Alternate knee to chest
     B. Alternate left arm, right leg extension
     C. Pelvic tilt
     D. Curl up
     E. Squat

175. Recent studies have indicated that a decrease in injuries to joints has resulted from increased
     A. Weight.
     B. Flexibility.
     C. Food supplements.
     D. Calcium intake.
     E. Frequency of exercise.

176. One of the major advantages of isokinetic resistance exercise over isotonic resistance exercise when rehabilitating an injured athlete is
     A. A constant amount of resistance delivered through the full range of motion.

     B. Increased range of motion.
     C. Hyperplasia of muscle fibers.
     D. Decreased lactic acid accumulation.
     E. The safety, because the resistance will not exceed the amount of force that can be produced.

177. Which modality uses the minimal effective dose (MED) test?
     A. Ultraviolet
     B. Infrared
     C. Vapocoolants
     D. Hyperbaric
     E. Paraffin

178. What is the biomechanical rationale for the use of a forearm strap in the treatment of lateral epicondylitis of the elbow?
     A. Increase the mechanical advantage of the flexor-pronator muscle groups
     B. Provide improved stability to the proximal radioulnar joint
     C. Reduce the range of the humeroulnar joint
     D. Modify the pull of the extensor-supinator mechanism at its origin
     E. Change the angle of pull at the origin of the flexor muscle group

179. What structure's collagen fibers are oriented to the line of functional force and are in the most regular formation?
     A. Fascia
     B. Tendon
     C. Ligament
     D. Bone
     E. Skin

180. Which of the following information should be recorded in the **objective** portion of an athlete's SOAP note?
     A. "The athlete does not want to return to athletics."
     B. "The athlete will regain 10 degrees of flexion in 2 weeks."
     C. "The athlete's swelling has decreased 0.5 inch."
     D. "The athlete is not putting maximal effort into the rehabilitation plan."
     E. "The athlete displays 1+ instability of the MCL."

181. Which of the following terms describe(s) the type of exercise in which the speed of exercise remains the same while the tension developed is maximal over the full range of motion?
    A. Plyometric
    B. Isotonic
    C. Isometric
    D. Eccentric
    E. Isokinetic

182. An athlete receiving continuous ultrasound application can safely experience which one of the following sensations?
    A. A mild muscle contraction
    B. "Pins and needles" sensation
    C. An intense muscle contraction
    D. A mild sensation of warmth
    E. An intense sensation of warmth

183. When designing a rehabilitation program for elbow lateral epicondylitis, the major muscles that need to be strengthened are
    A. Radial flexor of the wrist, ulnar flexor of the wrist, and the flexors of the fingers.
    B. Radial extensor of the wrist, ulnar extensor of the wrist, and abductor of the great toe

    C. Radial flexor of the wrist, ulnar flexor of the wrist, and rounded pronator.
    D. Radial extensor of the wrist, ulnar extensor of the wrist, and the brachioradialis.
    E. Radial extensor of the wrist, ulnar extensor of the wrist, and rounded pronator.

184. A 19-year-old wrestler is suffering from an open wound on the forearm. The wound has the classic signs associated with local inflammation and infection. If the athlete is placed on medication by the physician, the medication prescribed would likely be
    A. A corticosteroid.
    B. An anesthetic.
    C. A beta blocker.
    D. An analgesic.
    E. An antibiotic.

185. Increased pigmentation is a physiological effect of
    A. Cold.
    B. Heat.
    C. Ultrasound.
    D. Ultraviolet.
    E. Radiant energy.

ANSWERS FOR SAMPLE WRITTEN QUESTIONS

DOMAIN IV: TREATMENT, REHABILITATION, AND RECONDITIONING

1. B	18. C	35. B	52. D	69. C
2. C	19. C	36. A	53. B	70. A
3. A	20. A	37. A	54. A	71. D
4. A	21. B	38. D	55. C	72. C
5. C	22. C	39. D	56. D	73. D
6. E	23. C	40. C	57. A	74. C
7. D	24. A	41. A	58. C	75. D
8. A	25. B	42. C	59. B	76. A
9. E	26. D	43. C	60. A	77. B
10. A	27. E	44. C	61. B	78. D
11. E	28. A	45. B	62. A	79. B
12. C	29. C	46. A	63. D	80. A
13. D	30. A	47. D	64. C	81. B
14. E	31. A	48. A	65. A	82. C
15. C	32. A	49. E	66. E	83. C
16. D	33. B	50. C	67. A	84. A
17. A	34. B	51. D	68. B	85. D

86. B	106. E	126. E	146. B	166. D
87. D	107. C	127. A	147. E	167. D
88. B	108. C	128. A	148. C	168. B
89. A	109. B	129. C	149. A	169. C
90. E	110. B	130. B	150. B	170. A
91. B	111. D	131. D	151. D	171. A
92. B	112. D	132. B	152. B	172. B
93. C	113. A	133. D	153. A	173. A
94. A	114. B	134. C	154. C	174. B
95. A	115. A	135. A	155. C	175. B
96. C	116. A	136. C	156. C	176. E
97. B	117. C	137. D	157. C	177. A
98. D	118. B	138. A	158. A	178. D
99. B	119. A	139. B	159. C	179. B
100. A	120. A	140. D	160. B	180. C
101. A	121. A	141. E	161. C	181. E
102. E	122. A	142. E	162. A	182. D
103. A	123. C	143. D	163. D	183. D
104. C	124. B	144. E	164. A	184. E
105. B	125. D	145. E	165. B	185. D

SAMPLE WRITTEN QUESTIONS

DOMAIN V: ORGANIZATION AND ADMINISTRATION

1. The primary responsibility of the athletic trainer is
   A. Taping.
   B. Emphasizing curative practices.
   C. Keeping the training room clean.
   D. Caring for and prevention of athletic injuries.
   E. Hydrating the athletes.

2. What is the name of the organization that is responsible for improving the standards of athletic training?
   A. American College of Sports Medicine
   B. American Medical Association
   C. National Athletic Trainers Association
   D. Council on Medical Education and Hospitals of the American Medical Association
   E. National Strength and Conditioning Association

3. A meeting with your team physician(s) before the season could best be used to
   A. Get to know each other.
   B. Let the physician know what you expect from him or her.
   C. Present a plan for health care to athletes and refine it.
   D. Tell the coach how to handle the athletic training aspects of the job.
   E. Discuss the health concerns of the athletes.

4. What four areas should be developed with guidelines before the start of a season?
   A. Emergency plan, immediate care of injuries, rehabilitation program, general policies
   B. Treatment procedures, surgical priority, general policies, ambulance requirements
   C. First aid principles, specific exercises, general policies, physician concern
   D. Physician responsibilities, flexibility programs, general policies, hospital responsibilities
   E. General policies, strength and conditioning, coaching concern, classroom responsibilities

5. When an individual fails to act in a reasonable and prudent manner or, as is sometimes stated, "with due care," it is an example of
   A. Tort.
   B. Negligence.
   C. Liability.
   D. Felony.
   E. Prudence.

6. Which of the following is not a necessary or functional area of an athletic training room?
   A. Taping area
   B. Hydrotherapy area
   C. Storage area
   D. Shower
   E. Office

7. Hydrotherapeutic modalities should be cleaned at least
   A. Yearly.
   B. Once a month.
   C. Once a day.
   D. Once a week.
   E. Twice a week.

8. A junior high school athlete requests that her medical records be sent to a local outpatient clinic. Before you release this information to the clinic, you must
   A. Obtain a signed release from the athlete.
   B. Obtain a signed release from the athlete's parents or guardian.
   C. Obtain a signed release from the team physician.
   D. Obtain a signed release from the athlete's primary coach.
   E. Do nothing. No release is needed if the records are given to the athlete.

9. A piece of equipment costing $4000 and having a life span of 3 or more years is an example of
   A. Expendable supplies.
   B. Nonexpendable supplies.
   C. Capital supplies.
   D. Big-ticket supplies.
   E. Overhead supplies.

10. A professional scout contacts you about the medical records of a college senior who is a football player. What procedure must you follow before releasing this information?
    A. Provide the scout with the necessary information and note it in the athlete's file.
    B. Copy all records and supply copies to the scout.
    C. Refer the scout to the sports information director.
    D. Obtain a signed release form from the athlete.
    E. Refer the scout to the team physician.

11. Although securing goods and services through competitive bidding is generally considered desirable for an athletic department, direct purchase would be preferable to bidding when
    A. The goods or services are known to be available from only one source.
    B. The buyer has had satisfactory dealings with a specific supplier.
    C. There are a great many suppliers of the item requested.
    D. Some of the suppliers dealt with previously have been unsatisfactory.
    E. Only one supplier is available in the immediate area.

12. An employer can be held liable for the acts of his or her employees through
    A. Contributory negligence.
    B. Vicarious liability.
    C. Charitable immunity.
    D. Good Samaritan clause.
    E. Assumption of risk.

13. Regarding athletic facilities, which of the following is not the responsibility of the athletic trainer?
    A. Informing the coaching staff if the grass is too high.
    B. Ensuring that the blocking sled is properly padded.
    C. Reporting and/or correcting uneven playing surfaces.
    D. Ensuring that goal posts are properly padded.
    E. Informing the coaching staff that the practice field was just fertilized.

14. The essentials of a useful inventory in any well-managed athletic training department should include a/an
    A. Biannual check of all nonexpendable equipment.
    B. Annual check and estimate of both expendable and nonexpendable equipment.
    C. Careful listing of nonexpendable equipment lost or misplaced during the year.
    D. Careful listing of all expendable equipment lost or misplaced during the year.
    E. Evaluation of the expendable equipment most frequently used during the course of a year.

15. An established emergency care plan is an essential element in an institution's policy and procedure manual. Which of the following is not essential in an emergency care plan?
    A. The format for writing SOAP notes.
    B. A rehearsal plan.
    C. Designating a person to make the telephone call to activate the emergency medical services.
    D. Identifying the individuals possessing keys to areas such as the athletic training room, padlocks on gates, and so on.
    E. The type of information to be given over the telephone to emergency personnel.

16. An athletic trainer who uses a therapeutic modality in a contraindicated manner could be found guilty of which type of negligence?
    A. Malfeasance
    B. Misfeasance
    C. Nonfeasance
    D. Breach of duty
    E. Tort

17. Which of the following would not be considered a method of developing physician rapport?
    A. Present a professional image
    B. Develop a situation in which the physician feels like he or she is part of the program
    C. Set up a list of guidelines for the physician
    D. Have a meeting before the season to develop guidelines
    E. Encourage open communication between the physician and the athletes

18. Which of the following is not a duty of an athletic trainer?
    A. Work with doctor
    B. Fill in for nurse
    C. Supervise the athletic training room
    D. Administer first aid
    E. Supervise student athletic trainers

19. Medical diagnoses
    A. Are routinely made by athletic trainers.
    B. May only be made by a licensed physician.
    C. Cannot be used as evidence in a liability case.
    D. Are legal wrongs that legal scholars have difficulty defining.
    E. Do not apply to injuries sustained in sports.

20. It is important to develop a level of _____ between the coach and the physician.
    A. Professional integrity
    B. Mutual respect and awe
    C. Mutual admiration and suspicion
    D. Mutual confidence and trust
    E. Approval and affection

21. If the coach and/or parent feels more should be done regarding an injured athlete he or she should
    A. Seek a physician who will recommend what he or she thinks is necessary.
    B. Ask an athletic trainer from a nearby college as to what should be done.
    C. Ask the physician for a consultation with a specialist.
    D. Do what the coach thinks is best.
    E. Ask a student athletic trainer what he or she thinks is best.

22. What aspect of the athletic program must be met before the athlete is issued equipment?
    A. Fitness test
    B. Orthopedic examination
    C. Strength test
    D. Physical examination
    E. Mental examination

23. The key to successful relationships with the coach, coworkers, athletes, and administration is to
    A. Make sure they understand your position.
    B. Communicate well.

C. Just do your job well.

D. Give sound advice to others about how to do their jobs well.

E. Come to work on time.

24. How many square feet are considered adequate for an athletic training room?

A. 400–600

B. 700–900

C. 1000–1200

D. 1300–1500

E. 1550–1750

25. Someone who has a fractured jaw should be referred to a/an

A. Dentist.

B. Ophthalmologist.

C. Orthopedic surgeon.

D. Oral surgeon.

E. Plastic surgeon.

ANSWERS FOR SAMPLE WRITTEN QUESTIONS

DOMAIN V: ORGANIZATION AND ADMINISTRATION

1. D	6. D	11. A	16. B	21. C
2. C	7. C	12. B	17. C	22. D
3. C	8. B	13. A	18. B	23. B
4. A	9. C	14. B	19. B	24. C
5. B	10. D	15. A	20. D	25. D

SAMPLE WRITTEN QUESTIONS

DOMAIN VI: PROFESSIONAL DEVELOPMENT AND RESPONSIBILITY

1. All of the following are acceptable methods for the certified athletic trainer to obtain continuing education credit, except

A. Attending a district athletic training symposium in the district in which you are a member.

B. Attending a district athletic training symposium in a district in which you are not a member.

C. Attending the National Athletic Trainers Association (NATA) national symposium.

D. Reading articles and completing continuing education unit quizzes in approved journals.

E. Serving as an athletic trainer for a district all-star game.

2. All of the following are acceptable methods for the certified athletic trainer to obtain continuing education credit except

A. Serving as a panelist at a clinical symposium where the primary audience is allied health-care professionals.

B. Completing college coursework in administration.

C. Completing home study courses offered by a facility listed in the NATA Board of Certification (BOC)-approved provider directory.

D. Obtaining cardiopulmonary resuscitation recertification.

E. Providing an interview on athletic training for the local newspaper.

3. The branch of the federal government that approves and regulates the use of many therapeutic modalities is the

A. Underwriter's Laboratory (UL).

B. National Operating Committee on Standards for Athletic Equipment (NOCSAE).

C. Federal Trade Commission (FTC).

D. Food and Drug Administration (FDA).

E. American Physical Therapy Association (APTA).

4. The primary tasks of an entry-level athletic trainer have been identified by
   A. The NATABOC Role Delineation Study.
   B. The NATA Education Council's Competencies in Athlete Training.
   C. NATABOC Standards of Practice.
   D. The NATA Code of Ethics.
   E. The Commission for the Accreditation of Allied Health Education Programs.

5. Which of the following is not a responsibility of the athletic trainer?
   A. Maintaining documentation
   B. Implementing rehabilitation programs
   C. Preventing injuries
   D. Dispensing medications
   E. Educating coaches, athletes, and parents

6. Which of the following organizations accredits entry-level athletic training education programs?
   A. Commission on Accreditation of Allied Health Education Programs (CAAHEP)
   B. American Academy of Sports Medicine (AASM)
   C. American Physical Therapy Association (APTA)
   D. NATA Research and Education Foundation (NATA-REF)
   E. NATA Board of Certification (NATABOC)

7. Each of the following statements about continuing education requirements for NATABOC-certified athletic trainers is true **except**
   A. Each time you become recertified in cardiopulmonary resuscitation, continuing education units (CEUs) are awarded.
   B. The accumulation of CEUs must occur within a 3-year period.
   C. CEUs may be obtained by attending workshops and seminars.
   D. Becoming involved in the NATABOC certification testing program can count toward CEUs.
   E. First aid is **not** a continuing education requirement.

ANSWERS FOR SAMPLE WRITTEN QUESTIONS

DOMAIN VI: PROFESSIONAL DEVELOPMENT AND RESPONSIBILITY

1. E	3. D	5. D	6. A	7. A
2. E	4. A		

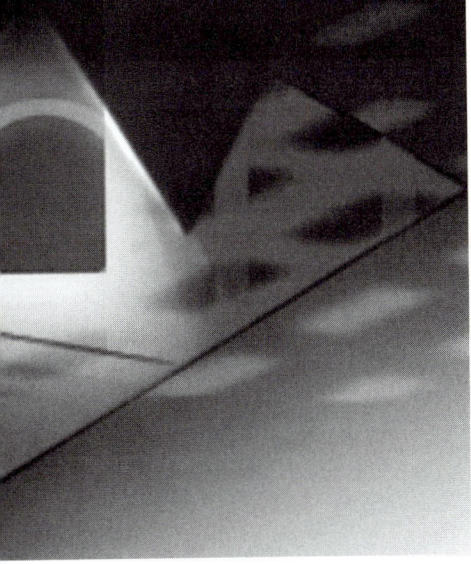

CHAPTER 7

The Simulation Examination

▓ SIMULATION EXAMINATION INFORMATION

The problems in this section of the examination are designed to test your decision-making ability in athletic training. To take this section of the examination, you will need the latent-image pen and the *Simulation Answer Booklet*. Although this study guide contains four sample simulation questions, the actual examination will have eight such problems. The correct answers and point values for each response are provided at the end of this chapter.

Time Allowed

You will have 2.5 hours to complete the simulation portion of the examination.

Instructions

Read the opening scene, which provides the introductory facts with which you will work. Read this situation, and all subsequent sections, carefully and follow the directions provided. Some sections ask for more than one response. **Choose all responses that you believe are relevant to the circumstances given.** If you fail to choose a response that should have been highlighted, you will not receive full credit for the section. Similarly, if you highlight a response that should not have been chosen, points will be deducted from your score.

In each section, choices appear in a random order. The response you choose will provide you with specific information and the results of your decisions, or

it will provide you with specific instructions. Use the information and results to determine your course of action for the next section. If you are given additional instructions, follow them exactly. Failure to do so will result in deductions from your score and may make it impossible to complete the problem correctly.

> ### Helpful Hints
>
> If you are one of those individuals who reveals too much, start by revealing the answers that give you additional information (i.e., information answers) and not those that are "action items." Even if you know you are going to reveal more than one answer, reveal the "information items" first.
>
> For example, if you do not know which to reveal first: "Take the athlete's pulse" or "Place the athlete on a backboard," then choose "Take the athlete's pulse" because that could give you more information about the scenario. Placing an athlete on a backboard (an action item) may also be necessary but more than likely will not give you additional information about the scenario.

Continue to work through the problems section by section until you uncover the response "End of Problem" with your latent-image pen. Some problems may not contain this response. If not, it will be noted in the section instructions for that particular problem. When you uncover this response, **do not go back into the problem and uncover additional responses.** This is not likely to improve your score and may result in penalties.

SIMULATION EXAMINATION SAMPLE QUESTIONS

SAMPLE PROBLEM 1

OPENING SCENE

A volleyball player has injured her left ankle during practice. You have completed your evaluation, and you suspect a moderate second-degree lateral ankle sprain.

Go to Section A

Section A

Immediately after your evaluation, you will do which of the following? (Choose only those actions that you have reason to believe are essential to the resolution of the case.)

1. Tape her ankle securely and see if she can finish practice.
2. Apply ice to the left ankle.
3. Have the athlete walk the injury off.
4. Write a note to excuse her from classes tomorrow.
5. Apply a compression wrap to the injured ankle.

Go to Section B

Section B

Volleyball practice is over now, and you and the athlete are in the athletic training room. The amount of swelling has increased since you evaluated the injury, and the athlete cannot bear weight without pain. Indicate your actions at this time. (Choose only those actions that you have reason to believe are essential to the resolution of this case.)

6. Secure, measure, and instruct the athlete in the use of crutches.
7. Call the coach to tell her the swelling has increased.
8. Give the athlete a warm whirlpool treatment.

Go to Section C

Section C

The team physician sees the athlete and diagnoses the injury as a moderate second-degree lateral ankle sprain. The physician does not apply a splint or cast but instructs the athlete to continue using crutches as long as the weight bearing causes pain. The physician refers the athlete back to you with proper instructions. What action will you take next? (Choose only those actions that you have reason to believe are essential to the resolution of the case.)

9. Instruct the athlete to continue the ice treatments for the rest of the day until she goes to sleep.
10. Instruct the athlete to use a heating pad on her ankle while she sleeps.
11. Instruct the athlete to call the coach to tell her what the doctor said.
12. Uncover response 12.

■ *End of Sample Problem 1*

SAMPLE PROBLEM 2

OPENING SCENE

You are the athletic trainer in charge of a district track meet. While you are observing the finals of the high hurdles, the public address announcer asks you to report to the pole vault pit area because an athlete has been injured.

Go to Section A

Section A

With the information now available to you, which of the following would you do? (Choose only those that you consider to be essential to the situation at this point.)

1. Instruct a meet official to halt all running and field events immediately.
2. Ask the athlete if he has pain anywhere other than in the area already noted.
3. Determine if the athlete's vault has been declared legal.
4. Ask the athlete where the pain is.
5. Ask the athlete if he has ever pole-vaulted before.
6. Ask the athlete to get up and walk.
7. Ask the athlete to explain what happened.
8. Check the athlete for severe bleeding.

9. On the way to the pole-vault area, ask witnesses what has happened.

10. As you approach the athlete, note the position of his body.

11. On your way to the pole-vault area, stop and tell a student athletic trainer to call for an ambulance.

12. Determine the level of consciousness of the athlete.

13. Go immediately to your first aid station and get ice bags and a penlight.

14. Ask the athlete to roll over.

Go to Section B

Section B

With the information you now have available, which actions would you perform at this time? (Choose only those that you have reason to believe are particularly relevant to the case at this point.)

15. Ask the athlete if he has ever injured his elbow before.

16. Check for Kehr's sign.

17. Palpate left acromioclavicular joint.

18. Check athlete's grip strength, bilaterally.

19. Check dorsalis pedis pulse and sensation in both feet.

20. Visually examine the left knee for swelling, bleeding, and deformity.

21. Ask the athlete if he has ever injured either knee before.

22. Ask the athlete if he felt the knee give way on him.

23. Palpate abdomen for rigidity.

24. Ask the athlete if he has ever injured his shoulder before.

25. Help the athlete get up and walk off the runway so the event can begin again.

26. Ask the athlete if he heard or felt a snap or pop.

27. Visually examine the right knee for swelling, bleeding, and deformity.

Go to Section C

Section C

With the information you now have available, which actions would you perform at this time? (Choose only those that you have reason to believe are particularly relevant to the case at this point.)

28. Palpate the right ankle for deformity.

29. Palpate the lateral aspect of the right knee for point tenderness and swelling.

30. Palpate the popliteal area of the right knee for tenderness and swelling.

31. Palpate the cervical spine.

32. Palpate the anterolateral joint line of the right knee for point tenderness and swelling.

33. Palpate the right piriform insertion area for tenderness and swelling.

34. Palpate the right quadriceps insertion, the patella, and the patellar tendon for tenderness and swelling.

35. Palpate the right olecranon process.

36. Palpate the left ankle for deformity.

37. Palpate the right knee for deformity.

38. Palpate the quadriceps and the hamstring muscles for spasm or deformity.

39. Palpate the anteromedial joint line of the right knee for point tenderness and swelling.

40. Check the athlete's pupillary responses with a penlight.

41. Palpate the medial aspect of the right knee for point tenderness and swelling.

42. Palpate the left knee for deformity.

Go to Section D

Section D

At this point in your examination, which of the following actions would you perform? (Choose only those that you have reason to believe are particularly relevant to this case at this time.)

43. Warn the athlete that he might have an injury that will require surgery.

44. Perform the Yergason test.

45. Ask the athlete to attempt to vault again.

46. Perform a varus and valgus stress test to the left knee, with knee flexed at 20 degrees.

47. Check the active range of abduction of the right knee.

48. Perform a varus and valgus stress test to the right knee, with knee flexed at 20 degrees.

49. Ask the athlete to run.

50. Administer two aspirins to the athlete to reduce his pain and help calm him.

51. Ask the athlete to execute a full squat.

52. Perform the Apley scratch test.

53. Check the active range of flexion of the right knee.
54. Test the knee for passive hyperextension.
55. Perform a varus and valgus stress test to the left knee fully extended.
56. Perform a varus and valgus stress test to the right knee fully extended.
57. Check the active range of motion of the left knee.
58. Perform the patellar apprehension test on the right knee.
59. Perform the Lachman drawer test or the anterior drawer test on the right knee.
60. Perform the Lachman drawer test or the anterior drawer test on the left knee.
61. Check the active range of adduction of the right knee.
62. Perform the McMurray meniscal test on the right knee.

Go to Section E

Section E

It has been 2½ hours since the injury. You have taken the athlete to the athletic training room and have given proper immediate care to the injury. The team physician is coming to examine the athlete after finishing surgery. In the meantime, the physician has asked you to reexamine the injury. What actions would you now take? (Choose only those actions that you have reason to believe are particularly relevant to the case at this point.)

63. Check for Tinel's sign.
64. Tell the athlete he has a minor injury.
65. Perform the McMurray meniscal test on the right knee.
66. Tell the athlete that he has an injury that will require surgery.
67. Perform the Lachman drawer test or the anterior drawer test on the right knee.
68. Ask the athlete to perform a full squat.
69. Perform the Thomas test.
70. Measure the circumference of the right thigh for atrophy.
71. Perform the Lachman drawer test or the anterior drawer test to the left knee.
72. Perform a varus and valgus stress test to the left knee.
73. Perform a varus and valgus stress test to the right knee.

74. Check the active range of motion of the right knee.
75. Perform the patellar apprehension test on the right knee.
76. Ask the athlete to bear weight.
77. Check for a hematoma in the right lower leg.
78. Palpate the right knee for tenderness and deformity.
79. Visually examine for swelling.
80. Passively move the right knee from 0-degree extension to 130-degree flexion.

Go to Section F

Section F

Based on the findings of your examination, what is your impression of the nature of this injury? (Choose only one.)

81. Anterior cruciate ligament injury.
82. Lateral collateral ligament injury.
83. Patellar subluxation.
84. Jumper's knee.
85. Medial collateral ligament injury.
86. Lateral meniscus injury.
87. Medial meniscus injury.

■ *End of Sample Problem 2*

SAMPLE PROBLEM 3

OPENING SCENE

A high school football player collapses during contact drills. Your sling psychrometer readings taken before practice were: dry bulb temperature of 88°F and 80% relative humidity.

Go to Section A

Section A

You have performed an initial assessment (a primary survey), and the athlete has an airway, is breathing, and has a pulse. As you begin your focused history and physical examination (secondary survey), the athlete spontaneously regains consciousness. With the information now available to you, you will do which of the following? (Choose only those that you consider to be essential to the situation at this point.)

1. Take a history from the athlete.
2. Retract the athlete's facemask.

3. Apply a cervical collar to stabilize the athlete's head and neck.
4. Take the athlete's radial pulse.
5. Activate emergency medical services (EMS).
6. Take the athlete's blood pressure.
7. Take the athlete's respiration rate.
8. Have two other players pick the athlete up and carry him into the locker room.
9. Evaluate the reaction of the athlete's pupils.
10. Evaluate the athlete's skin for color and moistness.
11. Apply inline, manual stabilization to stabilize the athlete's head and neck.
12. Evaluate pulses, motor function, and sensation in each extremity.
13. Draw-up a tube of blood for evaluation of the athlete's blood glucose level at a later time.
14. Ask the athlete's coach what the athlete was doing when he collapsed.
15. Go inside to the file cabinet and refer to the athlete's medical history provided during the preparticipation physical examination.

Go to Section B

Section B

You and the athlete are now in the air-conditioned locker room. You have determined that the athlete does not have a cervical spine injury, and you have removed the cervical collar. You have also ruled out diabetes and seizure based on past medical history. You suspect heat-related illness. You have removed the athlete's equipment. The athlete is complaining of a headache, hunger, and thirst. What will you do next? (Choose only those that you have reason to believe are particularly relevant to the case at this point.)

16. Give the athlete aspirin.
17. Take the athlete's core temperature.
18. Remove the athlete's clothes and/or equipment.
19. Apply fans and mist bottles.
20. Provide the athlete with oral fluids.
21. Have the athlete take a warm shower.
22. Have the athlete go home and rest.
23. Give the athlete salt pills.
24. Have the athlete return to practice.
25. Leave the athlete and go back outside to notify the coach as to his condition.

26. Send someone out to get the athlete something to eat.
27. Give the athlete an oral glucose solution to treat his diabetes.
28. Determine the athlete's mental status and whether he is alert and oriented.

Go to Section C

Section C

It is 10 minutes later, and the athlete complains of lightheadedness. When you attempt to converse with him he is obviously confused. He begins to shiver from the fans. He begins to cramp in both lower legs and in his abdomen. What actions would you now take? (Choose only those that you have reason to believe are particularly relevant to the case at this point.)

29. Take his core temperature again.
30. Cover him with a blanket to stop his shivering.
31. Massage his cramps with Flexall-454®.
32. Apply ice packs to the area of cramps and try to stretch them.
33. Apply ice packs to the groin, axilla, and neck.
34. Try to force oral fluids.
35. Activate EMS.
36. Give him muscle relaxants that were prescribed for one of the coaches.
37. Ask the athlete more questions.

Go to Section D

Section D

Based on the findings of your examination, what is your impression of the nature of this injury? (Choose only one.)

38. Epilepsy
39. Diabetic coma
40. Heat stroke
41. Concussion
42. Insulin shock
43. Heat exhaustion
44. Heat syncope
45. Fractured cervical vertebrae

■ *End of Sample Problem 3*

SAMPLE PROBLEM 4

OPENING SCENE

A high school football player collapses during contact drills. Your sling psychrometer readings taken before practice were: dry bulb temperature of 88°F and 80% relative humidity.

Go to Section A

Section A

You have performed an initial assessment (a primary survey), and the athlete has an airway, is breathing, and has a pulse. As you begin your focused history and physical examination (secondary survey), the athlete spontaneously regains consciousness. With the information now available to you, you will do which of the following? (Choose only those that you consider to be essential to the situation at this point.)

1. Take a history from the athlete.
2. Retract the athlete's facemask.
3. Apply a cervical collar to stabilize the athlete's head and neck.
4. Take the athlete's radial pulse.
5. Activate emergency medical services (EMS).
6. Take the athlete's blood pressure.
7. Take the athlete's respiration rate.
8. Have two other players pick up the athlete and carry him into the locker room.
9. Evaluate the athlete's pupil reaction.
10. Evaluate the athlete's skin for color and moistness.
11. Apply inline, manual, stabilization to stabilize the athlete's head and neck.
12. Evaluate pulses, motor function, and sensation in each extremity.
13. Draw up a tube of blood for evaluation of the athlete's blood glucose level at a later time.
14. Ask the athlete's coach what the athlete was doing when he collapsed.

15. Go inside to the file cabinet and refer to the athlete's medical history provided during the preparticipation physical examination.

Go to Section B

Section B

You and the athlete are now in the air-conditioned locker room. You have determined that the athlete does not have a cervical spine injury, and you have removed the cervical collar. You have also ruled out diabetes and seizure based on past medical history. The athlete is complaining of a headache. What will you do next? (Choose only those that you have reason to believe are particularly relevant to the case at this point.)

16. Give the athlete aspirin.
17. Take the athlete's core temperature.
18. Remove the athlete's equipment.
19. Apply fans and mist bottles.
20. Provide the athlete with oral fluids.
21. Have the athlete go home and rest.
22. Give the athlete salt pills.
23. Have the athlete return to practice.
24. Send the athlete home with instructions to not sleep.
25. Leave the athlete and go back outside to notify the coach as to his condition.
26. Give the athlete an oral glucose solution to treat his diabetes.
27. Determine the athlete's mental status and whether he is alert and oriented.

Go to Section C

Section C

It is 10 minutes later, and the athlete complains of lightheadedness. When you attempt to converse with him he is obviously confused. What actions would you now take? (Choose only those that you have reason to believe are particularly relevant to the case at this point.)

28. Take his core temperature again.
29. Provide oral fluids.
30. Call his parents to come pick him up.
31. Activate EMS.
32. Ask the athlete more questions.

Go to Section D

Section D

Based on the findings of your examination, what is your impression of the nature of this injury? (Choose only one.)

33. Epilepsy
34. Diabetic coma

35. Heat stroke
36. Concussion
37. Insulin shock
38. Heat exhaustion
39. Airway obstruction
40. Fractured cervical vertebrae

■ *End of Sample Problem 4*

SIMULATION EXAMINATION ANSWER KEY

(+) = Indicated Response
(0) = Neutral Response
(–) = Contraindicated Response

SAMPLE PROBLEM 1

Section A

Information gained from the stem:

- The athlete has a moderate sprain of the left ankle.
- The lateral ligaments have been injured.

1. (–) The information in this question's opening scene should have alerted you to the fact that this athlete's immediate return to competition is doubtful. Note the opening scene's reference to "a moderate second-degree ankle sprain." The fact that this injury occurred during practice further reduces the urgency of the athlete's immediately returning to competition.

2. (+) This is part of the proper protocol in the immediate treatment of traumatic injuries.

3. (–) The information presented in the opening scene of this question should alert you to the fact that walking off this injury is not an appropriate action. Note the close similarity between this question and question 1. The responses to number 1 and number 3 should have alerted you not to select the other response.

4. (0) Although this action does not cause further injury to the athlete, it is an unnecessary step at this point. Additionally, many institutions would not accept such an excuse from an athletic trainer.

5. (+) This action is clearly indicated because it is an essential element in the immediate care of an injury.

Section B

Information gained from the stem:

- The amount of swelling has increased.
- She is unable to walk on the ankle.

6. (+) The scenario of Section B indicates that the athlete's condition has worsened and clarifies the point that the athlete is unable to bear weight. Of the three actions listed, this one is the most clearly indicated.

7. (0) This action neither hurts nor helps the athlete's condition. Because the coach is not in her office, the disposition of the athlete should be relayed at a later time.

8. (–) The use of both whirlpool and heat are contraindicated in an acute injury. Whirlpools are avoided in acute conditions because the limb is placed in a dependent position, and the agitation of the water can potentially increase the inflammatory response. The use of heat is contraindicated because it increases the inflammatory response.

Section C

Information gained from the stem:

- Your initial impression of this injury has been confirmed by a physician (second-degree inversion ankle sprain).
- Because the ankle has not been placed in a splint or cast, it is physically capable of being treated.
- The athlete is to continue with the treatment of your choice until the athlete returns to full weight-bearing status.

9. (+) Ice application is still the accepted protocol at this time because it decreases the inflammatory process, decreases pain and muscle spasm, and limits the amount of secondary hypoxic injury.

10. (–) Because the inflammatory process is still active, heat application is not the accepted protocol at this time.

11. (0) This is a proper administrative procedure. Unfortunately, you are unable to contact the coach at this time.

SAMPLE PROBLEM 2

Section A

Information gained from the stem:

- You know only that an athlete has been injured at the pole-vault pit. The purpose of this section is for you to determine the nature and extent of the injury.

1. (0) This action would be appropriate only if the athlete were lying in the track or other location where further harm could result.

2. (+) This step is necessary to rule out injury to other body parts. Although not scored in this manner, this question should be asked after questions 4 and 7.

3. (0) Whether or not the athlete's vault was legal has little bearing on the athlete's injury.

4. (+) This step is needed to determine the location of the injury. You should note that the injury is to the right knee and/or thigh.

5. (0) This question is not needed at this time.

6. (–) Because you have not completed your evaluation, it is not prudent to have the athlete attempt to walk at this time.

7. (+) This question is needed to ascertain the mechanism of the injury. The logical progression would be to uncover this response after uncovering response 4.

8. (0) This response, although the proper action, is considered to be neutral because it does not specifically relate to the injury at hand.

9. (–) The best practice is to arrive at the scene before asking your questions. By stopping and asking questions, you are wasting valuable time, especially if this injury is life-threatening.

10. (+) This should be the first response uncovered in this section because it can be performed before asking any questions.

11. (–) Calling an ambulance before establishing the severity of the injury is a premature action.

12. (+) This action should coincide with, or immediately follow, response 10. The response indicates that the athlete is in pain and moving; therefore, the neurological functions are also intact.

13. (–) It is more appropriate to send someone to get ice bags when the need has been established rather than delay your response time. Additionally, it is more efficient to keep a penlight with you rather than going and getting one each time it is needed.

14. (–) Response 10 indicates that the athlete is lying face up, and response 4 indicates that this is a knee injury. It is not necessary to have the athlete roll over at this time.

Section B

Information gained from the previous section (section A):

- The athlete is conscious and breathing.
- The athlete has injured his right knee.
- The mechanism of injury occurred before the jump.

Information gained from the section B stem:

- The stem indicates that you are to continue with your evaluation.

15. (–) It has been established that this athlete suffered an injury to the right knee. Therefore, evaluating the elbow is inappropriate and unnecessary. Make certain that you carefully read the response before highlighting it.

16. (–) The Kehr sign is indicative of a ruptured spleen, and, based on the responses of sections A and B, you would have no reason to suspect an injury to the spleen.

17. (–) It has been established that this athlete suffered an injury to the right knee. Therefore, evaluating the left acromioclavicular joint is inappropriate and unnecessary. Make certain that you carefully read the response before highlighting it.

18. (–) The athlete is suffering from an injury to the right knee. At this point, your evaluation should focus on this body area.

19. (0) This action is most appropriate after a fracture or dislocation in the lower extremity to ensure that blood is still reaching the distal extremity. Although there is no indication that the trauma is this severe, you are erring on the side of caution.

20. (+) Bilateral comparison is essential when performing the observation phase of injury evaluation. This allows for a determination of any gross deformity, swelling, or discoloration.

21. (+) It is important to note whether the involved knee has been injured previously to distinguish between new and preexisting dysfunction. It is important to establish whether the uninvolved

knee has been previously injured so that bilateral comparisons are not clouded by other conditions.

22. (+) This question is part of this history-taking process and is used in determining the nature of the injury.

23. (−) This action is useful in determining abdominal injury. However, at this point, you should have no reason to suspect such pathology.

24. (−) It has been established that this athlete suffered an injury to the right knee. Therefore, evaluating the left shoulder is inappropriate and unnecessary. Make certain that you carefully read the response before highlighting it.

25. (−) At this point you have not completed your evaluation of the injury, so moving the athlete is premature.

26. (+) Questioning the athlete is an integral part of the history-taking process.

27. (+) Before palpating the injured area, the athletic trainer should inspect the site for any obvious deformity. Ideally, response 20 should be the next response you highlight.

Section C

Information gained from the previous section (section B):
- The athlete was injured as a result of his right knee "giving way."
- The right knee has a small amount of swelling but no other obvious deformities.

Information gained from the section C stem:
- The stem indicates that you are to continue with your evaluation.

28. (−) The right knee is the injured body area. Palpating the right ankle is not a necessary action.

29. (+) Palpation is a necessary element in the evaluation of an athletic injury. This response should have been uncovered with responses 30, 32, 34, 37, 39, and 41 to completely palpate the knee.

30. (+) Palpation is a necessary element in the evaluation of an athletic injury. This response should have been uncovered with responses 29, 32, 34, 37, 39, and 41 to completely palpate the knee.

31. (−) Because the athlete has not complained of cervical pain or numbness in the extremities, this action is unnecessary.

32. (+) Palpation is a necessary element in the evaluation of an athletic injury. This response should have been uncovered with responses 29, 30, 34, 37, 39, and 41 to completely palpate the knee.

33. (−) The piriform muscle, located in the hip, is very difficult to palpate. The evaluation should be limited to the knee.

34. (+) Palpation is a necessary element in the evaluation of an athletic injury. This response should have been uncovered with responses 29, 30, 32, 37, 39, and 41 to completely palpate the knee and adjacent structures.

35. (−) Because the elbow is not the injured area, there is no need to palpate the olecranon process.

36. (−) This action is not appropriate because it is the right knee that is injured.

37. (+) Palpation is a necessary element in the evaluation of an athletic injury. This response should have been uncovered with responses 29, 30, 32, 34, 39, and 41 to completely palpate the knee.

38. (0) The musculature is intact, and muscle guarding has not occurred at this time. If spasm were present, this could "mask" future ligamentous tests.

39. (+) Palpation is a necessary element in the evaluation of an athletic injury. This response should have been uncovered with responses 29, 30, 32, 34, 37, and 41 to completely palpate the knee.

40. (0) This is not a step in evaluating an injured knee.

41. (+) Palpation is a necessary element in the evaluation of an athletic injury. This response should have been uncovered with responses 29, 30, 32, 34, 37, and 39 to completely palpate the knee.

42. (+) It is necessary to palpate the uninvolved body part to compare these findings with that of the injured limb.

Section D

Information gained from the stem:
- The stem indicates that you are to continue with your evaluation.
- There is "mild tenderness" on the medial aspect of the right knee.
- The athlete is point tender around the anteromedial joint line.
- There is a small amount of swelling around the anteromedial joint line.

43. (−) The athletic trainer is not qualified to determine surgical injuries. Such a statement will unnecessarily alarm the athlete.

44. (−) The Yergason test is used to evaluate the stability of the long head of the biceps muscle of

the arm. This test is not necessary for a knee injury.

45. (–) Because your evaluation of the injury is incomplete, this action is premature.

46. (+) It is important to compare the results of ligamentous stress tests of the injured body part to the noninvolved side.

47. (–) The knee does not actively abduct.

48. (+) Varus stress is used to evaluate the integrity of the lateral collateral ligament, and valgus stress applied at 20 degrees of flexion is used to evaluate the deep fibers of the medial collateral ligament. Because these tests are negative, the likelihood of injuring these structures is reduced.

49. (–) Because the severity of this athlete's injury has not been established, functional tests such as running should be avoided.

50. (–) Aspirin would do little to calm an injured athlete.

51. (–) The results from the active range of motion tests of the involved and uninvolved knees should have alerted you to the fact that this motion could not be accomplished without pain.

52. (–) The Apley scratch test is used to evaluate active abduction, internal rotation, and external rotation of the humerus. This test is not required when evaluating a knee.

53. (+) Active range of motion is necessary when evaluating a knee injury.

54. (+) The highlighted response indicates that the injured knee hyperextends when compared with the uninvolved knee. This result should be noted for future reference in the problem.

55. (+) It is important to compare the results of ligamentous stress tests between the injured body part and the noninvolved side.

56. (+) Varus stress checks the integrity of the lateral collateral ligament; valgus stress applied when the knee is in complete extension checks the integrity of the superficial and deep fibers of the medial collateral ligament. Because these tests are negative, the likelihood of injuring these structures is reduced.

57. (+) The results of the test for active range of motion of the right knee compared with that of the left knee indicate that the injured limb is lacking 20 degrees of flexion.

58. (+) The patellar apprehension test is used to evaluate a dislocating or subluxating patella.

59. (+) The anterior drawer test and the Lachman test are used to evaluate the integrity of the anterior cruciate ligament. The positive results of these tests should be noted for future reference.

60. (–) The tests for anterior ligament instability are negative on the uninvolved knee, thus reinforcing the findings of response 59.

61. (–) The knee does not actively adduct.

62. (+) The McMurray test is used to detect lesions to the medial or lateral menisci.

Section E

Information gained from the previous section (section D):

- The injured knee (right knee) is lacking 20 degrees of flexion.
- The right knee hyperextends relative to the left knee.
- An anterior drawer and/or Lachman test elicited positive results, indicating anterior cruciate ligament laxity.
- All other tests (valgus stress, varus stress, McMurray test, and the apprehension test) were negative.

Information gained from the section E stem:

- Two and one half hours have elapsed since the injury.
- You have treated the athlete with "proper immediate care," consisting of ice, compression, and elevation.
- You have been asked to reevaluate the athlete.

63. (0) The Tinel sign is used to evaluate hypersensitive nerves.

64. (–) The severity of the injury has not been established at this time. Because the physician is on the way to evaluate this injury, statements such as this are best left unsaid.

65. (+) Although the McMurray test for meniscal lesions was negative the first time, it is a good idea to completely reevaluate the knee at this point. Note that the limited amount of knee flexion will make performing the McMurray test difficult.

66. (–) Athletic trainers are not qualified to differentiate between surgical and nonsurgical injuries. Leave this type of decision to the physician.

67. (+) Although this test is now negative, recall that it was positive the first time you performed it. The negative result found during the reevaluation is most likely because of the onset of muscle spasm and/or muscle guarding.

68. (–) If you uncovered response 51 in section D, you noted at this point that this action resulted

in a great deal of pain. If you did not uncover this response earlier, you will note that the athlete is lacking the full range of motion in the right knee.

69. (–) The Thomas test is used to evaluate flexion contractures of the hip. This test is not necessary when evaluating an acute knee injury.

70. (0) The atrophy process begins after as little as 24 hours of immobilization. No injury-related atrophy of the quadriceps group would be noted at this point.

71. (+) It is important to compare the results of ligamentous stress to the opposite body part.

72. (+) This action is done to compare the results of the injured body part with the uninjured part.

73. (+) Although this test was negative during your immediate evaluation, it is proper procedure to perform a complete knee evaluation during the subsequent examination.

74. (+) Note that the athlete has lost an additional 15 degrees of flexion and now actively hyperextends 15 degrees. The lack of active flexion could be related to pain and muscle spasm; the increased hyperextension could be indicative of increased anterior cruciate ligament laxity.

75. (+) This response indicates that you are performing a thorough examination of the knee.

76. (–) Based on your findings in this and previous sections, it should be apparent that this action is unnecessary.

77. (0) It is possible that blood and edematous fluid have drained down to the lower extremity. If the limb was elevated as a part of the "proper immediate care," the likelihood of a hematoma forming in this area is decreased.

78. (+) As found during the previous palpation, the athlete is point tender over the anteromedial joint line.

79. (+) Despite the ice, compression, and elevation, the knee continues to swell. This is usually indicative of a moderate to severe injury.

80. (–) This action is inappropriate because the athlete is limited to 95 degrees of active flexion. Active range of motion should always be tested before passive range of motion.

Section F

Information gained from the previous section (section E):

- Although the anterior drawer test and Lachman test were initially positive, they now produce negative results. This is most probably caused by muscle spasm.

- The amount of swelling continues to increase.
- The athlete has lost an additional 15 degrees of active flexion secondary to swelling and muscle spasm.
- The athlete's right knee hyperextends 15 degrees.

Information gained from the section F stem:

- You are asked to arrive at a conclusion regarding the nature of this injury.

81. (+) This is the correct conclusion based on the information gained in the five sections of this problem. The positive anterior drawer test and Lachman test, knee hyperextension, lack of flexion, and swelling are all indicative of an injury to the anterior cruciate.

82. (–) Because the varus stress test was negative in both your initial and your follow-up evaluation, it is unlikely that this structure was damaged.

83. (–) The athlete did not display a hypermobile patella when the apprehension test was performed.

84. (–) Jumper's knee (infrapatellar tendinitis) is an injury marked by an insidious onset.

85. (–) Because all valgus stress tests were negative, it is unlikely that this structure was damaged.

86. (–) A positive McMurray's test eliciting pain along the lateral joint line would have indicated this type of injury.

87. (–) A positive McMurray's test that elicits pain along the medial joint line would have indicated this type of injury.

SAMPLE PROBLEM 3

Section A

Information gained from the stem:

- The athlete is a football player participating in contact drills.
- The ambient environment is hot and humid.

1. (+) A history is always one of the first and most important parts of an examination. In this case, the fact that the athlete is confused is an important finding.

2. (–) This need has not yet been established. Retracting or removing a football player's facemask is indicated once a spinal injury is suspected and the need for transportation has been determined.

3. (0) A need for this has not been clearly indicated, but applying a cervical collar to the ath-

lete initially could be considered a cautious, but appropriate, response at this time. At this point a head or spine injury has not been ruled out. It is known that the athlete is participating in a collision sport and that he is confused and unable to respond appropriately. This should be done after response 11.

4. (+) Obtaining a heart rate is an important part of the physical examination.

5. (–) Calling an ambulance before establishing the nature or severity of the injury or illness is, in this case, premature. There is nothing, at this point, to indicate a life-threatening or severe condition.

6. (0) Blood pressure is probably the least important vital sign to assess in this situation because it is time consuming and requires additional equipment that you may not have readily available. In addition, you should know that the athlete has a systolic blood pressure of at least 90 mmHg because you were able to obtain a radial pulse.

7. (0) Respiration rate is also not very important in this situation. The important part is that the athlete is breathing, which is something that you established in your initial assessment. The rate itself may not tell you much because the athlete was just exercising in the heat.

8. (–) The athlete may have a neck injury. A need for moving the player has not yet been determined, and other potential injuries have not been ruled-out at this time.

9. (+) Evaluating pupil reaction is an important part of the physical examination, particularly when a head injury is suspected. The fact that the pupils were equal, round, and reactive to light does not rule out a head injury, but it is a good indication that, if a head injury is present, it is not severe.

10. (+) Evaluating skin condition is an important part of the physical examination, particularly when heat-related illness is suspected. The fact that the skin is red, warm, and moist does not tell you much, given that the athlete was just exercising in the heat. The skin being moist does not rule out heat-related illness, but it is a good indication that if heat-related illness is present, it is not severe (i.e., less likely that it is heat stroke).

11. (+) Initially, inline cervical stabilization should be applied, until a spine injury has been ruled out or the need for a cervical collar has been determined. A spine injury cannot be ruled out before evaluating the athlete's pulses, motor, and sensation. It is known that the athlete is participating in a collision sport and that he is confused and unable to respond appropriately.

12. (+) Evaluating the athlete's pulses, motor function, and sensation in all four extremities is an important part of the neurological examination when a spine injury is suspected. The fact that the athlete had strong pulses and good motor function and was able to detect sharp and light sensation in each extremity does not rule out spine injury but is a good indication that if an orthopedic spine injury is present, it is likely not severe and/or does not involve the spinal cord.

13. (–) Evaluating blood glucose can be a nice diagnostic procedure, particularly if the athlete is a known diabetic and a hand-held glucometer is readily available. However, these have not been established at this time. Furthermore, it is not appropriate for an athletic trainer to draw blood for evaluation of the athlete's blood glucose level at a later time.

14. (+) Because the athlete is confused and was unable to respond appropriately to your questions earlier, it is a good idea to interview bystanders or family. This should have been done after performing response 1.

15. (–) It is not appropriate to leave the athlete at this time.

Helpful Hints

Most of the questions you will receive during the actual certification examination are based on fact or are a universally accepted standard or practice in athletic training, or both. However, with the simulation questions, not every athletic trainer may agree that an action is necessary or appropriate, and they most certainly will not always agree with the sequence in which the steps should be taken (i.e., answers revealed). Therefore, it is likely that the way you have been taught to deal with this simulation may not be the same as the answers provided. Do not be alarmed.

Section B

Information gained from the previous section (section A):

- The athlete's pupil reaction is normal.
- The athlete's skin is red, warm, and moist.
- The athlete has a history of heat-related illness.
- The athlete has an altered mental status.

Information gained from the stem:

- This is not a cervical spine injury, diabetic emergency, or seizure event.
- The athlete has a headache and is thirsty and hungry.
- The athlete has stopped practicing, he has been removed from the heat to a cool environment, and his equipment and some of his clothes have been removed.
- Heat-related illness is suspected.

16. (–) In general, athletic trainers are not permitted to dispense medication. Furthermore, aspirin can mask symptoms and alter the sequelae of injury. This mistake is not life threatening but was a very poor choice.

17. (+) Obtaining an athlete's core temperature is an important part of the physical examination and is the single greatest indicator of heat-related illness. The fact that his temperature was 105°F confirms any suspicions of heat-related illness.

18. (+) Removing the athlete's clothes exposes more skin to the environment and allows for more efficient cooling.

19. (+) Using fans and mist bottles is a very effective method of cooling. This should be done after the athlete's clothes are removed.

20. (+) Providing cool oral fluids is indicated in cases of suspected heat-related illness, and many forms of heat-related illness are related to, or exacerbated by, dehydration.

21. (–) This is absolutely contraindicated. When heat-related illness is suspected, the objective is to cool the body. A warm shower can elevate the athlete's core temperature even more.

22. (–) This action is contraindicated. It is inadvisable to send the athlete home without first treating his condition.

23. (–) This action is contraindicated. Salt pills are no longer used in the treatment of heat-related illness.

24. (–) This action is wrong. Placing the athlete back in a hot environment and returning him to activity would certainly elevate his core temperature and could result in heat stroke.

25. (–) It is inadvisable to leave the athlete at this time. Although it is proper to advise the coach as to the athlete's condition, it is not required at this point in your immediate management of this illness and/or injury.

26. (–) Although hunger can be an indication of hypoglycemia, it has been established that this is not a diabetes-induced illness.

27. (–) Oral glucose was administered, although there is no indication for this treatment at this time.

28. (–) The athlete knows who he is and where he is but does not know what day it is or how he got to the locker room. This indicates an altered mental status.

Section C

Information gained from the previous section (section B):

- His temperature is 105°F, indicating heat-related illness.

Information gained from the stem:

- You have been treating the athlete for heat-related illness.
- The fans are providing cooling.
- Cramps, which were not present earlier, have now started.
- The athlete is now lightheaded.

29. (+) His core temperature is now 107°F. This indicates that the athlete's body is not responding to cooling techniques. Despite removing the athlete from the heat and spending at least 15 minutes cooling him, his core temperature continues to rise to dangerous levels.

30. (–) Shivering can be prompted by malfunctions in the hypothalamus (during extreme elevations in temperature) or by aggressive cooling of the skin (which is what is being done with the fans and misting), but core temperature is the more important factor. Despite the athlete's shivering, his core temperature is 107°F, and he is obviously suffering from extreme heat-related illness. Aggressive cooling is indicated in an attempt to dissipate body heat. Any efforts to retain body heat are expressly contraindicated.

31. (–) Although massage may be indicated for muscle cramps, no counterirritants should be used.

32. (+) Massage is indicated for muscle cramps. Ice massage is a good technique for reducing the cramps and for cooling the body.

33. (+) Applying ice over the major blood vessels in the body is a valid attempt to cool the body.

34. (+) Although the athlete vomited the first time this was attempted, it is worth trying again. The ingestion of cool fluids can treat the dehydration accompanying the heat-related illness, and even if the fluids are not kept in the body,

they act to cool the body core when they are ingested.

35. (+) This action is now indicated. The fact that the athlete is not responding to cooling techniques and is developing additional signs and symptoms (cramps and lightheadedness) indicates that his condition is deteriorating. This is now becoming a medical emergency. The athlete is at risk of damaging his internal organs and brain with the high fever. Immediate transportation, intravenous therapy by the EMS personnel, and continual care and evaluation in an emergency medical receiving facility are indicated.

36. (–) This action is never permitted. It is illegal to prescribe or dispense medication without a license, and it is illegal and improper to dispense one person's medication to another.

37. (+) Performing a "serial assessment," "ongoing assessment," or "continuous assessment" is appropriate to determine whether the athlete's condition is improving or worsening. In this case, discovering that "the athlete is more confused than before" is a clear indication that his condition is deteriorating.

Section D

Information gained from the previous section (section C):

- Core temperature continues to increase, despite cooling methods.
- The athlete's mental status is worsening.
- The athlete is cramping and vomiting.
- Ice has been applied.
- EMS has been activated.

38. (–) Although the medical history was missing from the file, this athlete was not known to have epilepsy and had not had a witnessed seizure. Epilepsy was ruled out in the section B stem.

39. (–) Although thirst and altered mental status can be an indication of diabetic coma, a result of hyperglycemia, it can also be the result of dehydration. Diabetes-related illness was ruled out in the section B stem.

40. (+) Heat stroke is the correct response. The severity of thermal injury (increased core temperature) and altered mental status make this a medical emergency.

41. (–) Although concussion or other mild brain injury was suspected because of the athlete's altered mental status and participation in contact drills, it was partially eliminated in response 9.

42. (–) Although hunger can be an indication of insulin shock, a result of hypoglycemia, it can also be the result of not eating or of strenuous physical activity. Diabetes-related illness was ruled out in the section B stem.

43. (–) Heat exhaustion may have been the correct response early in the scenario, but by the end of the problem, the deteriorating athlete was in heat stroke.

44. (–) Heat syncope is a very mild form of heat-related illness. The information from this question would indicate a more severe form of heat-related illness.

45. (–) A fractured cervical vertebra was suspected because of the athlete's participation in contact drills, but it was partially eliminated by response 12 and was ruled out in the section B stem.

Helpful Hints

Because the responses to this question may not have been considered universally accepted standards or practices in athletic training, this question is useful in demonstrating different options. This question in particular was made even more difficult because heat-related illness is not experienced as commonly in some parts of the country as in others. Because of this, some individuals are not as familiar with all of the latest techniques or information for recognizing and treating heat-related illness. Moreover, the individuals who are more comfortable and familiar with heat-related illness are more likely to treat mild to moderate heat-related illness themselves, whereas those who are less familiar and comfortable with recognizing the severity and urgency of the illness might opt for a more prompt referral. This question should not be thought of as a bad question (because different individuals may treat it differently) but rather as a good demonstration of how each of us should progress through the problem. It will then make more sense on how you should progress through a more universally accepted problem, such as an ankle sprain.

SAMPLE PROBLEM 4

Section A

Information gained from the stem:

- The athlete is a football player participating in contact drills.
- The ambient environment is hot and humid.

1. (+) A history is always one of the first and most important parts of an examination. In this case, the fact that the athlete is confused is an important finding.

2. (–) This need has not yet been established. Retracting or removing a football player's facemask is indicated once a spinal injury is suspected and the need for transportation has been determined.

3. (0) A need for this has not been clearly indicated, but applying a cervical collar to the athlete initially could be considered a cautious, but appropriate, response at this time. At this point a head or spine injury has not been ruled out. It is known that the athlete is participating in a collision sport and that he is confused and unable to respond appropriately. This should be done after response 11.

4. (+) Obtaining a heart rate is an important part of the physical examination.

5. (–) Calling an ambulance before establishing the nature or severity of the injury and/or illness is, in this case, premature. There is nothing at this point to indicate a life-threatening or severe condition.

6. (0) Blood pressure is probably the least important vital sign to assess in this situation because it is time consuming and requires additional equipment that you may not have readily available. In addition, you should know that the athlete has a systolic blood pressure of at least 90 mmHg because you were able to obtain a radial pulse.

7. (0) Respiration rate is also not very important in this situation. The important part is that the athlete is breathing, which you established in your initial assessment. The rate itself may not tell you much because the athlete was just exercising in the heat.

8. (–) The athlete may have a neck injury. A need for moving the player has not yet been determined, and other potential injuries have not been ruled-out at this time.

9. (+) Evaluating pupil reaction is an important part of the physical examination, particularly when a head injury is suspected. The facts that the pupils were unequal and round and that the left pupil was slow to react to light are good indications of a head injury.

10. (+) Evaluating skin condition is an important part of the physical examination, particularly when heat-related illness is suspected. The fact that the skin is red, warm, and moist does not tell you much, given that the athlete was just exercising in the heat. The skin being moist does not rule out heat-related illness, but it is a good indication that if heat-related illness is present, it is not severe (i.e., less likely that it is heat stroke).

11. (+) Applying inline cervical stabilization should be performed initially, until a spine injury has been ruled out or the need for a cervical collar has been determined. A spine injury cannot be ruled out before evaluating the athlete's pulses, motor, and sensation. It is known that the athlete is participating in a collision sport and that he is confused and unable to respond appropriately.

12. (+) Evaluating the athlete's pulses, motor function, and sensation in all four extremities is an important part of the neurological examination when a spine injury is suspected. The fact that the athlete had strong pulses and good motor function and was able to detect sharp and light sensation in each extremity does not rule out spine injury but is a good indication that if an orthopedic spine injury is present, it is likely that it is not severe and/or does not involve the spinal cord.

13. (–) Evaluating blood glucose can be a precise diagnostic procedure, particularly if the athlete is a known diabetic and a hand-held glucometer is readily available. However, these have not been established at this time. Furthermore, it is not appropriate for an athletic trainer to draw blood for evaluation of the athlete's blood glucose level at a later time.

14. (+) Because the athlete was confused and unable to respond appropriately to your questions earlier, it is a good idea to interview bystanders or family. This should have been done after response 1.

15. (–) It is not appropriate to leave the athlete at this time.

Section B

Information gained from the previous section (section A):

- The athlete's pupil reaction is abnormal.
- The athlete's skin is red, warm, and moist.
- The athlete has a history of heat-related illness.
- The athlete has an altered mental status.

Information gained from the stem:

- This is not a cervical spine injury, diabetic emergency, or seizure event.
- The athlete has a headache.
- The athlete has stopped practicing, he has been removed from the heat to a cool environment, and his equipment and some of his clothes have been removed.
- Heat-related illness is suspected.

16. (−) In general, athletic trainers are not permitted to dispense medication. Furthermore, aspirin can mask symptoms and alter the sequelae of injury. This mistake is not life threatening but was a very poor choice.

17. (+) Obtaining an athlete's core temperature is an important part of the physical examination and is the single greatest indicator of heat-related illness. The fact that his temperature was 101°F may not tell you much because the athlete was just exercising in the heat.

18. (+) Removing the athlete's pads will make the athlete more comfortable, will facilitate your evaluation, and may signal the athlete that he is not ready to return to practice and that he may need some additional time to recuperate.

19. (−) There is no reason to use fans and mist bottles on this athlete.

20. (0) Providing oral fluids may have helped the athlete's thirst.

21. (−) This action is contraindicated. It is inadvisable to send the athlete home alone without first treating his condition.

22. (−) There is no reason to give salt pills to this athlete.

23. (−) Placing the athlete back in activity increases his risk for second impact syndrome.

24. (−) This action is contraindicated. It is inadvisable to send the athlete home without first treating his condition or releasing him to a qualified adult.

25. (−) It is inadvisable to leave the athlete at this time. Although it is proper to advise the coach as to the athlete's condition, it is not required at this point in your immediate management of this illness and/or injury.

26. (−) Oral glucose was administered, although there is no indication for this treatment at this time.

27. (−) The athlete knows who he is and where he is but does not know what day it is or how he got to the locker room. This indicates an altered mental status.

Section C

Information gained from the previous section (section B):
- His temperature is 101°F.

Information gained from the stem:
- The athlete is now lightheaded.
- The athlete is confused.

28. (+) The core temperature is now 99°F. This indicates that the athlete's body is cooling appropriately after being removed from a hot environment.

29. (−) Because the athlete vomited the first time and you do not suspect heat-related illness or dehydration, it is inadvisable to risk having him vomit again because vomiting can increase intracranial pressure.

30. (+) His parents cannot be reached.

31. (+) This action is now indicated. The fact that the athlete is more confused than before indicates that his condition is deteriorating. It is clear that this athlete needs medical attention, and because his parents cannot be contacted, it is now appropriate to transport the athlete to an emergency medical receiving facility for advanced care and evaluation.

32. (+) Performing a "serial assessment," "ongoing assessment," or "continuous assessment" is appropriate to determine whether the athlete's condition is improving or worsening. In this case, discovering that "the athlete is more confused than before" is a clear indication that his condition is deteriorating.

Section D

Information gained from the previous section (section C):
- Core temperature continues to decrease.
- The athlete's mental status is worsening.
- EMS has been activated

33. (−) Although the medical history was missing from the file, this athlete was not known to have epilepsy and had not had a witnessed seizure. Epilepsy was ruled out in the section B stem.

34. (−) Although thirst and altered mental status can be an indication of diabetic coma, a result of hyperglycemia, it can also be the result of dehydration. Diabetes-related illness was ruled out in the section B stem.

35. (−) Heat stroke was never a consideration.

36. (+) Concussion, or other brain injury, was suspected because of the athlete's altered mental status and participation in contact drills and because unequal and nonreactive pupils were revealed in question 9.

37. (−) Diabetes-related illness was ruled out in the section B stem.

38. (−) Heat exhaustion was ruled out with response 17 and again with response 28. An in-

ternal temperature of 101°F is normal for an athlete exercising in the heat while wearing protective equipment.

39. (–) Although an airway obstruction can cause changes in mental status, there was no indication that his airway was obstructed. It was re-vealed early in the scenario that he had an airway and was breathing and speaking.

40. (–) A fractured cervical vertebra was suspected because of the athlete's participation in contact drills, but it was partially eliminated by response 12 and was ruled out in the section B stem.

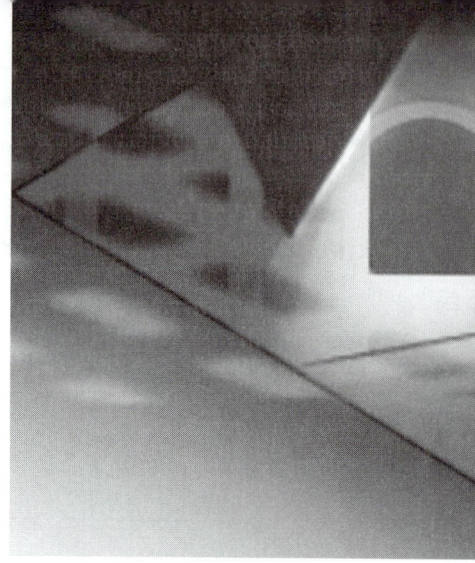

CHAPTER 8

The Practical Examination

◢ PRACTICAL EXAMINATION INFORMATION

This portion of the examination measures a candidate's ability to perform tasks (skills) that are described in the National Athletic Trainers Association Board of Certification (NATABOC) Role Delineation Study. Candidates are no longer required to "describe and demonstrate" a skill or procedure. The oral component ("describe") has been dropped from the examination's format.

The questions on the practical section of the examination are now task oriented. The actual examination contains 8 to 12 skills. These are situations that you could expect to encounter on a daily basis as a certified athletic trainer. The examiners' evaluation will be based solely on your demonstrations given in response to specific instructions, not on your apparent general knowledge and abilities.

Procedures When Performing During the Practical Examination Section

1. You will have a candidate's guide at your disposal and will be able to read the questions while the examiner reads them to you. You should read the question yourself because sometimes the examiner can misread the question. Also, you have a better chance of accurately processing the information if you see it in print.
2. There will be an audiotape recorder and three examiners: a model, a room captain, and an examiner in the room with you. The model **will not** verbally respond to your questions, but you should ask them anyway. Pretend that the model is an injured athlete and take control of the situation. You are in charge, so do what you need to do. You should treat the model the way you would have treated your own athlete the week before. Do not be afraid to touch the model or to ask questions or give directions. **The model will follow your directions.**

3. There will be a table of supplies for you to use. You may not bring any of your own materials, tools, or instruments into the examination room. Look at the table closely and take your time. While you are examining the materials, begin your mental imagery of how you might use the material. The supplies may be a clue to what skill you will have to demonstrate. There are no trick supplies or things on the table to distract you that you will not be asked to use. If you would have used a different material for the situation (such as a different sized elastic wrap, for example), mention that to the examiners and then proceed with the material that they have provided for you.

Helpful Hints

If the examiner asks you if you would like to have the question reread, your answer should be YES! An examiner does not ordinarily ask that question, unless you are doing something wrong. When the question is reread, pay close attention. The examiner is trying to help you get back on track and to answer the question differently.

4. The examiners have a short list of specific skills that you must demonstrate for each question. The examiners have the option of only "yes" or "no" for each specific task, so it is important that you be clear and demonstrate what they are asking. There is no penalty for going out of sequence. If you forget to perform a portion of your skill and there is time remaining, go back and complete your response.

5. To know how to respond to the questions, it is important to know how this section has evolved over the years. Questions used to be multiskilled; now they are very specific. For a long time, this was called the oral/practical section, and you were required to verbally describe everything that you were doing manually. It may help you to know that it is acceptable to explain what you are doing during the test (talk yourself through it).

6. You may ask how much time you have remaining.

To get an idea of what skills may be tested in this section, refer to the psychomotor skills that are described in the Role Delineation Study. Examples of the types of questions are provided in the following pages. It may be best to have a certified athletic trainer evaluate your performance in this portion of the study guide.

PRACTICAL EXAMINATION SAMPLE QUESTIONS

Instructions

At the beginning of this portion of the certification examination, the examiner will start the tape recorder and read a statement that will be similar to the following.

"On the table, there is a candidate's guide to the practical examination. It contains four situations that are encountered in the athletic training profession. You may refer to this guide as I read the instructions and situations to you. Do not turn the pages until given instructions to do so. Turn now to page 1. In this practical exam, you will be presented with several situations. For each situation, you will be instructed to explain and demonstrate specific athletic training techniques and procedures. You will be evaluated solely on your demonstrations given in response to specific instructions, not on your apparent general knowledge and abilities. The model is present only to allow you to demonstrate techniques and procedures. He or she will not give you any additional information regarding the situation but will follow your instructions. Do not expect the model to respond verbally to your questions. Take a moment to inspect the materials on the table. You may use any of the materials for your demonstration."

SAMPLE QUESTION 1

Evaluation of the Collateral Ligaments of the Finger

This situation allows you the opportunity to perform an examination that checks the integrity of the finger's medial and lateral collateral ligaments (radial and ulnar collateral ligaments). For purposes of this demonstration, please perform these tests on the proximal interphalangeal joint of the model's right index finger. You have 4 minutes to complete your response.

1. The candidate positions the model in an appropriate position.

   YES   NO

2. The candidate stabilizes the proximal phalanx of the finger being tested.

   YES   NO

3. The candidate grasps the middle phalanx of the finger being tested.

   YES   NO

4. The candidate positions the finger in its neutral position or flexed position but no more than 5 degrees.

   YES   NO

5. The candidate applies a force that stresses the medial (ulnar) collateral ligament of the proximal interphalangeal (PIP) joint.

   YES   NO

6. The candidate applies a force that stresses the lateral (radial) collateral ligament of the PIP joint.

   YES   NO

SAMPLE QUESTION 2

Demonstration of the Straight Leg Raise Test

This situation allows you to demonstrate your proficiency at performing the straight leg raising test to determine the possible irritation of the sciatic nerve. You have 4 minutes to complete your response.

1. The candidate positions the model in the supine position.

   YES   NO

2. The candidate stands at the side of the model being tested.

   YES   NO

3. The candidate grasps the leg being tested by the heel.

   YES   NO

4. The candidate extends the model's knee.

   YES   NO

5. The candidate flexes the model's hip while keeping the knee extended.

   YES   NO

SAMPLE QUESTION 3

Demonstration of Measuring Passive Range of Motion at the Knee

This situation allows you to demonstrate your skills in using a goniometer to measure passive knee flexion. You have 3 minutes to complete your response.

1. The candidate evaluates range of motion passively.

   YES   NO

2. The candidate correctly places axis of the goniometer on the lateral epicondyle.

   YES   NO

3. The candidate correctly places the proximal end of the goniometer along the lateral side of the femur.

   YES   NO

4. The candidate correctly places the distal end of the goniometer along the lateral side of the fibula.

   YES   NO

5. The candidate mentions that all measurements will be recorded for future reference.

   YES   NO

6. The candidate demonstrates or mentions that the measurements were taken bilaterally.

   YES   NO

SAMPLE QUESTION 4

Demonstration of Padding a Heel Spur

This situation allows you to demonstrate your skills in applying a pad to a heel spur. You have 2 minutes to complete your response.

1. The candidate cuts a round pad from felt.

   YES   NO

2. The candidate cuts a hole in the middle of the pad (to remove pressure).

   YES   NO

3. The candidate places pad on the heel correctly.

   YES   NO

4. The candidate applies tape neatly and wrinkle free to secure the pad.

YES   NO

5. The candidate completes the task under the allotted time.

YES   NO

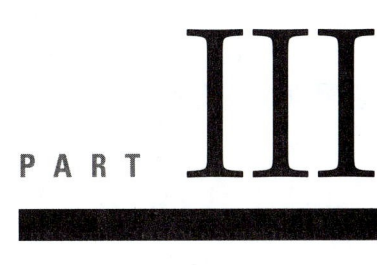

PART III

Appendices

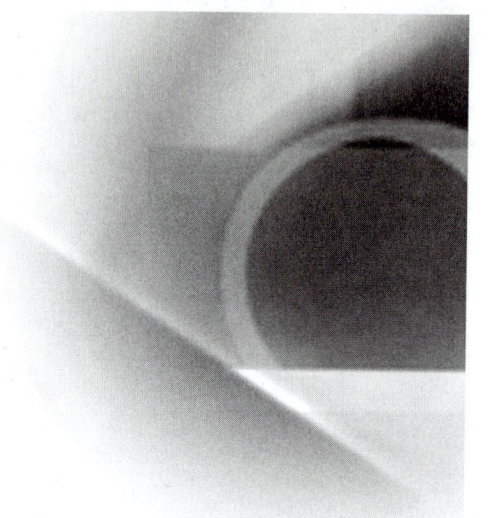

NATABOC Standards
for Athletic Training

Section 2

**STANDARDS FOR ATHLETIC TRAINING
SERVICE PROGAM**

The following are minimal standards. Each one is essential to the practice of athletic training. It is intended that these standards be used by administrators as well as by athletic training personnel in the development of their service programs, and to assess their effectiveness.

Standard 1: OBJECTIVES

Basic to the development of any program are its intended purposes. Objectives and applicable policies should be clearly outlined for each activity, such as: athletic treatment, education of personnel, supervision and interdisciplinary relations. The objectives of the service program should implement those of the institution itself.

Standard 2: PLANNING

Each objective should be supported by detailed plans for its implementation.

Standard 3: EVALUATION

Objective methods of data collection and analysis should be used in relation to each component of the program to determine the need for service, assess its effectiveness, and indicate a need for change.

Standard 4: TYPES OF SERVICES OFFERED

Athletic training is appropriately a health service offered under the direction of a physician or dentist for the prevention, immediate care, management/disposition and reconditioning of athletic injuries.

Standard 5: PERSONNEL

The service program should be directed by a NATABOC Certified Athletic Trainer who has met the qualifications established by the National Athletic Trainers Association Board of Certification, Inc.. Education, qualifications, and experience of all other personnel should meet existing standards, and should be appropriate to their duties.

Standard 6: FACILITIES AND BUDGET

Space, equipment, supplies, and a continuing budget should be provided by the institution, and should be adequate in amount, variety, and quality to facilitate the implementation of the service program.

Standard 7: RECORDS

Objective, permanent records of each aspect of the service program should: (1) indicate date, name of physician or dentist referral; (2) initial evaluation and assessment; (3) treatment or services rendered, with date; (4) dates of subsequent follow-up care.

Standard 8: REPORTS

Written reports on each aspect of the service program should be made annually.

Figure A–1 NATABOC Standards for Athletic Training Service Program.

Common Abbreviations and Terms

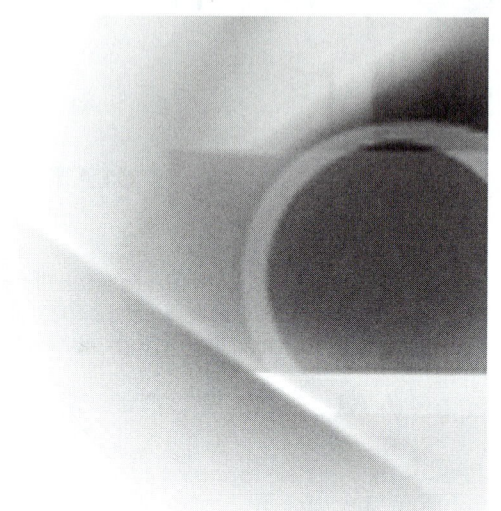

ADA – The Americans with Disabilities Act. The NATABOC complies with this regulation and offers reasonable accommodation because of disability.

Applicant – Any person who has requested an application for the certification examination from the NATABOC.

ATC – A certified athletic trainer. An allied health care professional who has fulfilled the requirements for certification as established by the NATABOC and has passed the certification examination administered by the NATABOC.

Basic requirements – The requirements that all applicants must fulfill before candidacy is granted by the NATABOC.

CAAHEP – The Commission on Accreditation of Allied Health Education Programs, the accrediting agency for entry-level athletic training educational programs.

CAHEA – The Committee on Allied Health Education and Accreditation. This accrediting committee of the American Medical Association (AMA) was the predecessor to CAAHEP.

Candidate – Any applicant whose application has been accepted and who is scheduled to take the NATABOC certification examination.

CAS – Columbia Assessment Services, the agency contracted by the NATABOC to administer and score the certification examination, now a part of CASTLE Worldwide Inc.

CCT – The Clinical Competency Test. This is the name used previously for the simulation section of the examination.

Certificant – An NATABOC-certified athletic trainer (i.e., an ATC).

CEU – Continuing education unit. ATCs must accumulate 80 CEUs for every 3-year period to maintain their certification.

Clinical hours – Any time (clock hours) spent under the direct supervision of an ATC. This is one of the basic requirements for candidacy. **Note:** Clinical hours may be obtained in a variety of settings.

CPR – Cardiopulmonary resuscitation. A valid certificate (card) in CPR is one of the basic requirements for candidacy.

Curriculum candidate – An NATABOC candidate who is a graduate of a CAAHEP-accredited athletic training educational program.

Curriculum route – An approved program of formal coursework and clinical hours that leads to NATABOC examination eligibility as a curriculum candidate.

EMT – Emergency medical technician. A valid EMT certificate is an acceptable alternative for satisfying the CPR requirement, which is one of the basic requirements for candidacy.

Formal coursework – Instruction of appropriate knowledge and skills in a structured classroom course.

Internship candidate – An NATABOC candidate, who is **not** a graduate of a CAAHEP-accredited athletic training educational program.

Internship route – An informal program consisting of certain formal courses and clinical hours that leads to

NATABOC examination eligibility as an internship candidate.

JRC-AT – The Joint Review Committee on Educational Programs in Athletic Training. The JRC-AT is the committee that recommends entry-level accreditation to CAAHEP and is also responsible for the approval of advanced-level athletic training educational programs.

NATA – The National Athletic Trainers Association.

NATA-PEC – The NATA Professional Education Committee. This committee preceded the Education Council.

NATABOC – The NATA Board of Certification, an autonomous certifying agency with the authority to grant the ATC credential.

NCCA – The National Commission for Certifying Agencies, the national agency that certifies the NATABOC.

NOCA – The National Organization for Competency Assurance. The NCCA is the accreditation body of NOCA.

Statistical Reliability of the NATABOC Certification Examination

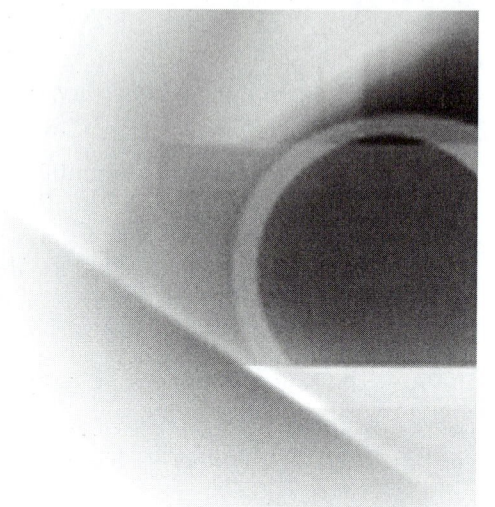

Originally written by

Said K Hayez, PhD,   George V. Richard, PhD,   and Ann Schulte, PhD

and modified for the 3rd edition

The National Athletic Trainers' Association (NATA), like many other professional associations, has been involved in certifying the level of performance of its members for many years. Certification is necessary to demonstrate that the individual worker is qualified to perform the required duties without threat of harm to the public. Many examinations have been developed to assess the minimum competence of entry-level workers in their profession. These examinations are called certification examinations.

The development of a certification examination is a long and complex process. It requires rigorous testing of the examination's validity or the ability of the test to measure that which it is supposed to measure. The validity of a certification examination involves the demonstration of at least two major qualities. First, the content of the examination must be shown to be job related. Second, the examination should cover areas in which lack of knowledge would cause harm to the public. These qualities make up some of the defining characteristics of what is called the content validity of the examination.

Another important characteristic in determining the quality of a certification examination concerns how reliable, or consistent, the examination is. Reliability is an index of how accurately the examination measures the candidate's skills. A test must be both valid and reliable for it to be considered a well-developed examination.

This report describes the development of the NATA Certification Examinations. Important topics discussed include the demonstration of the examination's validity and reliability. Also discussed is the method for determining the passing points for each section of the examination.

◼ DEVELOPMENT OF THE NATABOC CERTIFICATION EXAMINATION

The NATABOC has developed three sections to the examination that make up the certification process. These examinations have been developed to measure competence in three different areas of functioning. First, the NATABOC written examination assesses basic knowledge in the area of athletic training. The examination consists of 150 five-option multiple-choice questions from the six major content areas derived through the 1999 Role Delineation Study.

The second section of the examination, the practical examination, assesses critical skills in a more applied context by presenting a series of practical tasks and then asking candidates to manually demonstrate what course of action they would take. This test is designed to measure the candidate's performance skills.

In the third section of the NATABOC examination, the simulation section, the candidate's ability to evaluate a situation and make appropriate decisions is measured. Examinees are presented with eight written scenarios similar to those that could be encountered in actual practice. The examinees must then choose the action(s) they would take from among several alternatives.

The ability of the certification examinations to accurately assess entry-level performance is based in large part on their content validity. The process of validating the content of the NATABOC certification examination involved a rigorous, step-by-step process described in the following. Figure C–1 presents a diagram representing the steps in the content validation process.

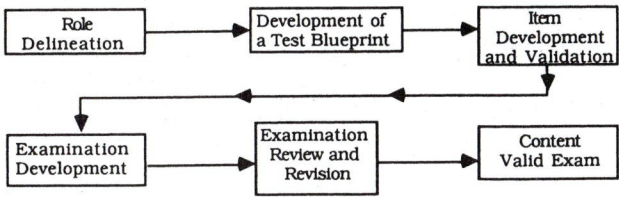

Figure C–1   Steps in constructing a content-valid examination.

1. **Role Delineation.** In the first step of the development of the NATABOC certification examination, a role delineation study was conducted. During this step, a special committee formed by the NATABOC classified the role of the athletic trainer in terms of the overall performance domains associated with the role. These performance domains were further broken down into more distinct tasks, knowledge, and skills required on the job. Figure C–2 provides a graphic representation of this breakdown.

   Using the data from this role delineation, a validation survey was developed and sent to 1000 athletic trainers. These athletic trainers rated each task, knowledge, and skill statement in the survey on several dimensions, including importance, criticality (or amount of possible harm that may occur to the public in the case of poor performance), and relevance for entry-level athletic trainers. The role delineation study was conducted in 1982, 1989, and 1999. It is continually updated when deemed necessary by the NATABOC.

2. **Development of a Test Blueprint.** In the next step, the results from both the role delineation study and the validation survey were used to develop a blueprint, or plan, for the certification examination. This blueprint was used as a guide for determining the content of the examination. Also, the information regarding the importance, harmfulness, and percentage of time devoted to each domain was translated directly into the percentage of items that should be included in the examination for each content area.

3. **Item Development.** The next stage in the development of the NATABOC certification examination was to develop items, or questions, that pertain to the areas of performance outlined in the test blueprint. All items for these examinations were written by individuals in the field of athletic training. Each item writer prepared several questions, then after undergoing training in editing, reviewing, and validating questions, the writers validated and classified each item into the appropriate content category and cognitive level based on the blueprint and on guidelines provided by Columbia Assessment Services, Inc. (CAS).

   Once the items were developed, reviewed, validated, and accepted, they were submitted to CAS, where they underwent a second psychometric and editorial review. After the second review, the final version of the item was entered into the NATA computerized item bank. These items could then be available for possible use in future NATABOC certification examinations.

4. **Examination Development.** Each examination is created by randomly selecting the appropriate number of items from each content area, as specified in the test blueprint. The items are then incorporated into a preliminary examination, and this examination is then reviewed by members of the NATABOC knowledgeable about each content area for any duplication of items or to evaluate whether any items cause any unforeseen problems. In essence, the item is again evaluated in terms of how psychometrically sound, fair, and content valid it is relevant to the whole examination.

5. **Examination Review and Revisions.** The NATABOC certification examinations (practical, written, and simulation examinations) are revised each year. These revisions are conducted to ensure that the examination continues to be a valid measure of candidates' abilities. All items from previous versions of the examinations are carefully reviewed and statistically analyzed. Using these analyses of statistical items, the inappropriate or questionable items are either revised or omitted from future examinations. When an item is removed, it is replaced with newly developed items. These new items are written by certified members of the NATA, validated (reviewed and analyzed) by at least three additional members and then edited, proofread, and psychometrically reviewed by CAS staff. Items that are accepted for inclusion in the examination must meet stringent validity requirements,

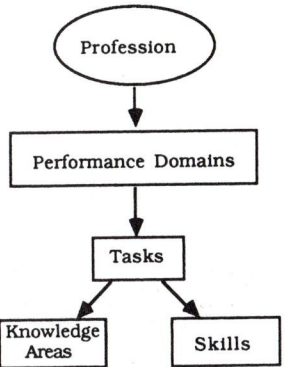

Figure C–2   The hierarchical arrangement of components in a role delineation study.

which include their degree of relevance to performance as a certified athletic trainer.

Each of the three examinations included in the NATABOC certification process has undergone developmental procedures similar to those outlined earlier. These procedures are necessary in the development of a content-valid certification examination. At each step in the process, a formal review is performed to determine the quality of the item and the examination. Based in part on these analyses, the psychometric quality of the examination is assured. As a result, the quality of the NATABOC certification examination can be considered to be of a high caliber.

RELIABILITY OF THE NATABOC CERTIFICATION EXAMINATION

In addition to content validity, a certification examination must also demonstrate that it is highly reliable, or consistent, in its measurement of entry-level performance. Examinees' scores should not be affected by factors such as testing conditions, different scoring standards used by different judges, or the particular version of an examination he or she happens to take. Theoretically, if the test is reliable, an examinee should be able to obtain the same or similar score at two different testing times or to be rated the same or similarly by two different raters on the examination. Statistical calculations of reliability estimates range from 0 to 1, with 1 indicating perfect reliability. A high reliability estimate for a certification examination, like that of the NATABOC, is generally considered by most authorities to be 0.80 or above.

One measure of reliability that is used in the NATABOC certification examination is called the Kuder-Richardson Formula 20 (KR-20), which is a measure of the internal consistency of the test. Internal consistency indicates the degree to which all of the questions on the NATABOC examinations measure common "characteristics" of the candidates. In other words, it provides us with an indication of the homogeneity of the examination or the ability of the test to measure a single content area. The better the examination is in measuring this single content area, the higher the reliability.

Internal consistency reliability estimates using the KR-20 method have been computed for both the practical and the written sections of the 1989 certification examination. The KR-20 calculation for the practical examination was 0.81, whereas the KR-20 estimate for the written examination was 0.88, suggesting high reliability.

Another type of reliability involves a comparison between the ratings of two or more judges on the performance of an examinee. This type of reliability is called inter-rater reliability. The practical examination requires the examinee to perform various skills while being rated by at least two judges. Inter-rater reliability is used to determine whether the ratings by these two judges are in agreement. The higher the agreement between the two judges, the higher the inter-rater reliability for the examination.

Over the years, the practical section has been revised considerably. The recent estimate of inter-rater reliability is 0.91, up approximately 10 points from previous versions of the examination. This suggests that questions on the practical section have been written in such a way that bias and error have little effect on ratings by independent judges.

If a test is reliable, one can expect that an examinee will obtain the same or similar score on the same examination at two different testing times. This type of reliability is called test-retest reliability. In 1989, CAS determined the test-retest reliability for the simulation section. The analysis was based on 110 candidates who had taken the same examination in January and again in May of 1988. The test-retest reliability for this group was 0.83, which indicated that the simulation section was reliable. This reliability index was based only on those candidates who failed the January 1988 simulation portion of the examination. The reliability index might have been higher if the test-retest analysis had been performed on the entire candidate population, encompassing candidates who passed as well as those who failed the examination.

RELATIONSHIPS BETWEEN THE WRITTEN, SIMULATION, AND PRACTICAL EXAMINATIONS

The three sections of the NATABOC certification examination have been developed to assess competence in separate areas of performance. As a result, the content of each of the three examinations is expected to differ markedly from the others. The method used to determine the amount of agreement among these three areas is called a correlation coefficient. The correlation can range from –1, which is a perfect negative correlation (meaning a high score on one examination corresponds to a low score on another examination), to +1, indicating perfect positive correlation (which means that a high score on one examination corresponds to a high score on another examination). When there is no correlation between two examinations, the correlation is 0. For the three sections of the NATABOC examination the correlations are expected to be low, because each examination measures separate areas of performance. In fact, this has been found to be generally true of the three sections of the NATABOC certification examination. The correlation

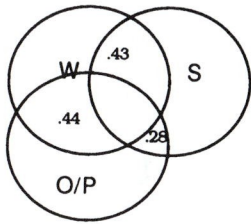

Figure C–3 Comparison of the intercorrelations among written (W), simulation (S), and practical (P) examinations.

between the written and the simulation sections is 0.43; the practical and simulation sections correlated 0.28, and the written and practical sections correlated 0.44. These correlations are considered low to moderate and indicate little overlap between the three examinations. Figure C–3 presents a graphic comparison of the amount of overlap among the examinations.

DETERMINING PASSING POINTS

Finally, a high-quality certification examination also has a defensible passing score. In other words, the cutoff score that separates examinees who pass from examinees who fail is determined in a systematic and reasonable way, rather than arbitrarily. There are several ways to set passing points. The method used by the NATABOC in its certification examinations is a criterion-referenced approach called the Modified Angoff Technique. The testing profession currently considers this technique to be one of the most defensible criterion-referenced methods available for setting passing points (Hayez, 1987). With this technique, the reviewers determine the minimum number of questions a competent examinee would be expected to pass. The passing point for the examination is based on the judgment, and it includes a statistical adjustment for testing error. This adjustment is provided to give the benefit of the doubt to examinees who score just below the level judged to be the minimal passing point by the reviewers. Because the NATABOC examination is revised each year, with questionable items replaced by newly developed items, the content and difficulty level of the examination changes. These revisions usually result in changes that affect the score necessary to pass. As a result, the passing point for each examination (i.e., written, simulation, and practical sections) must be adjusted.

SUMMARY

The procedures used to develop the NATABOC certification examination are accepted procedures for developing reliable and content-valid examinations. Each step in the test construction process is carefully documented. Through multiple reviews by content and psychometric experts and the use of stringent criteria, the validity of the test is assured. Also, reliability is important to assess the consistency of the test to measure examinees' skills accurately. Once the certification examination shows evidence of validity and reliability, it is important to use well-accepted procedures to set passing points. The Modified Angoff Technique, described earlier, is based both on judgments by members of the NATABOC and on statistical procedures to set the passing point for the NATABOC. As a result of all these safeguards, the NATABOC certification examination can be considered valid and reliable, with a sound method for determining passing points. With this process, the NATABOC is assured of the ability to accurately assess candidates' competence to carry out their assigned duties.

REFERENCES

American Psychological Association: Standards for Educational and Psychological Testing, Washington, DC, American Psychological Association, 1985.

Anastasi, A: Psychological Testing. Macmillan, New York, 1988.

Hayez, SK: An Introduction to Two Major Ways of Setting Passing Points. Report prepared for the National Athletic Trainers Association, 1987.

Hayez, SK: Overview of the National Board Examination for veterinary medicine. J Am Vet Med Assoc 188:807–810, 1986.

Hayez, SK, and Richard GV: An analysis of the inter-rater reliability of the Oral/Practical Examination of the National Athletic Trainers Association Certification Examination. Report presented to the Board of Certification of the National Athletic Trainers Association, 1989.

Kane, MT: The validity of licensure examinations. Am Psychol 37:911–918, 1982.

Shulte, A, and Hayez, SK: Content validation of the National Athletic Trainers Association Certification Examination. Report presented to the Board of Certification of the National Athletic Trainers' Association, 1988.

Schoon, CG, and Hayez, SK: The entry-level role of nursing home administrators. The Journal of Long-term Care Administration 15:15–18, 1987.

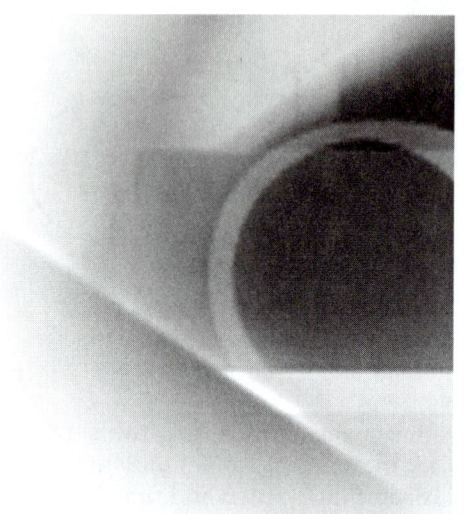

Appendix D

Study Sources and Reference List

The following is a reference list compiled by the National Athletic Trainers Association Board of Certification (NATABOC) for use in preparing for the certification examination and as documentation for correct answers. This list is not to be considered all-inclusive, and the most current edition is used as the reference.

ACSM's Exercise Management for Persons with Chronic Diseases and Disabilities, American College of Sports Medicine, Human Kinetics, 1997.

ACSM's Guidelines for Exercise Testing & Prescription, ed. 5. ACSM, Williams & Wilkins, 1995.

Agostini: Medical and Orthopedic Issues of Active and Athletic Women. Mosby, 1994.

American Academy of Orthopaedic Surgeons: Athletic Training & Sports Medicine, ed. 2. American Academy of Orthopaedic Surgeons, Chicago, 1991.

American College of Sports Medicine: Guidelines for Exercise Testing and Prescription. Lea & Febiger, Philadelphia, 1991.

American Red Cross: CPR for the Professional Rescuer. StayWell, 1993.

American Red Cross: Emergency Response. 1997.

American Red Cross: Standard First Aid Manual. 1991.

Anderson, M., and Hall, S: Sports Injury Management. Williams & Wilkins, 1995.

Anderson, M, & Hall, S: Fundamentals of Sports Injury Management. Williams & Wilkins, 1997.

Andrews & Harrelson: Physical Rehabilitation of the Injured Athlete. WB Saunders, Philadelphia, 1991.

Arnheim, DD, and Prentice, WE: Essentials of Athletic Training, ed. 4. WCB McGraw-Hill, 1999.

Arnheim, DD, and Prentice, WE: Principles of Athletic Training, ed. 10. McGraw-Hill, 2000.

Arky, Goodman, & Gillman: Therapeutics of Pharmacology. Medical Economics, 1988.

Baechle: Essentials of Strength Training & Conditioning. NSCA, Human Kinetics, 1994.

Baley, and Matthews: Law and Liability in Athletics, Physical Education, and Recreation. Allyn and Bacon Inc, 1984.

Bates: Guide to Physical Examination and History Taking, ed. 6. Lippincott, Philadelphia, 1995.

Baumgartner & Strong: Conducting & Reading Research in Health & Human Performance. 1998.

Berning & Nelson Steen: Sports Nutrition for the 90s: The Health Professional's Handbook. Aspen Publishers Inc, 1991.

Baumgartner & Jackson: Measurement for Evaluation in Physical Education & Exercise Science. WCB Brown & Benchmark, 1995.

Booher & Thibodeau: Athletic Injury Assessment, ed. 4. McGraw-Hill, 1994.

Ciccone: Pharmacology in Rehabilitation. Philadelphia, FA Davis.

Clarkson & Gilewich: Musculoskeletal Assessment: Joint Range of Motion and Manual Muscle Strength. Williams & Wilkins 1989.

Crosby, LA, and Lewallen, DG: Emergency Care & Transportation of the Sick & Injured, ed. 6. American Academy of Orthopaedic Surgeons, 1995.

Donatelli, RA: Physical Therapy of the Shoulder, ed. 2. Churchill-Livingstone, 1991.

D'Orazio, B: Back Pain Rehabilitation. Andover Medical Publishers, 1993.

Earle, MV: 1998–1999 NCAA Sports Medicine Handbook. NCAA 1998.

Fisher, AG, and Jensen, CR: Scientific Basis of Athletic Conditioning. Lea & Febiger, Philadelphia, 1990.

Fitzpatrick, et al.: Color Atlas and Synopsis of Clinical Dermatology: Common and Serious Diseases. McGraw-Hill Inc, 1992.

Fritz, S.: Mosby's Fundamentals of Therapeutic Massage. Mosby Lifeline, 1995.

Gallaspy and May: Signs & Symptoms of Athletic Injuries. Mosby, 1996.

Gallup, E.: Law and the Team Physician. Human Kinetics, 1995.

Greenberger and Hinthorn: History Taking and Physical Examination. Mosby, 1993.

Greenfield: Rehabilitation of the Knee: A Problem-Solving Approach. FA Davis, Philadelphia, 1993.

Griffin and Karselis: Physical Agents for Physical Therapists, ed. 2. Thomas Books, 1982.

Guyton: Medical Physiology. WB Saunders, Philadelphia, 1981.

Hales, D: An Invitation to Health. D. Brooks-Cole, 1997.

Hall, S: Basic Biomechanics. St. Louis, Mosby, 1995.

Hartley, A: Practical Joint Assessment: A Sports Medicine Manual. Mosby Year Book, 1990.

Heil: Psychology of Sport Injury. Human Kinetics, 1993.

Herbert, DL: Legal Aspects of Sports Medicine. Professional Reports Corporation, 1990.

Hertling, D, and Kessler, RM: Management of Common Musculoskeletal Disorders: Physical Therapy Principles & Methods, ed. 2, JB Lippincott, Philadelphia, 1990.

Hochschuler SH: The Spine in Sports, Hanley and Belfus, 1990.

Hoppenfeld: Physical Examination of the Spine & Extremities, Appleton-Century-Crofts, 1976.

Jenkins, DB: Hollinshead's Functional Anatomy of the Limbs & Back. WB Saunders, Philadelphia, 1990.

Jones & Bartlett: National Safety Council Bloodborne Pathogens. 1995.

Jordan, Tsaicis, and Warren: Sports Neurology. Aspen Publishers, 1989.

Journal of Athletic Training.

Kettenbach, G.: Writing SOAP Notes, ed. 2, FA Davis, Philadelphia, 1995.

Kendall, and Wadsworth: Muscles: Testing and Function. Williams & Wilkins, 1971.

Kibler, WB: The Sports Preparticipation Fitness Examination. Human Kinetics Books, Champaign, IL, 1990.

Kisner, C, and Colby, LA: Therapeutic Exercise: Foundations & Techniques, ed. 3, FA Davis, Philadelphia, 1996.

Knight, KL: Cryotherapy in Sport Injury Management. Human Kinetics, 1995.

Konin: Clinical Athletic Training. Slack, 1997.

Konin, JG, Wikstein, DL, and Isear, JS: Special Tests for Orthopedic Examination. Slack, Inc, 1997.

Kuland: The Injured Athlete, ed. 2. JB Lippincott, Philadelphia, 1988.

Magee, DJ: Orthopedic Physical Assessment, ed. 2. WB Saunders, Philadelphia, 1992.

Malone, T: Sports Injuries Management Series. Williams & Wilkins, Baltimore, 1990.

Mellion, MB: The Team Physician's Handbook. Hanley & Belfus, 1990.

Mellion, MB, et al: The Team Physician's Handbook, ed. 2., 1997.

McArkle, Katch, and Katch: Essentials of Exercise Physiology. Lee & Febiger (Williams & Wilkins), 1986.

McArdle, Katch, and Katch: Exercise Physiology: Energy, Nutrition and Human Performance, ed. 3. Lea and Febiger, Philadelphia, 1991.

Michlovitz, S: Thermal Agents in Rehabilitation, ed. 3. FA Davis, Philadelphia, 1996.

Moore, K: Clinically Oriented Anatomy. Williams & Wilkins, 1992.

NATA CEU Requirements & Appeal Process Brochure, NATA, 1997.

NATA Code of Ethics.

NATA News.

NATABOC Credentialing Brochure, 1998.

NATABOC Guidelines.

NATABOC Policies & Procedures.

NATABOC Recertification Guidelines, 1994–1996.

NATABOC: Role Delineation Study: Athletic Training Profession, ed. 4., Columbia Assessment Services, Inc, 1999.

O'Donahue: Treatment of Injuries to Athletes. WB Saunders, Philadelphia, 1984.

O'Keefe, M, et al: Emergency Care, ed. 8. Brady/Prentice Hall, 1998.

Orthopedic Physical Therapy for the Shoulder, Kelly and Clark, 1995.

Payton: Research: The Validation of Clinical Practice, ed. 3., FA Davis, Philadelphia, 1995.

Perrin: Athletic Taping & Bracing, Human Kinetics, 1995.

Perrin: Isokinetic Exercise and Assessment, Human Kinetics, 1993.

Peterson: Eat To Compete, 1996.

Pfeifer and Mangus: Concepts of Athletic Training, ed. 2. Jones & Bartlett, 1998.

Pollock and Wilmore: Exercise in Health and Disease, ed. 2. WB Saunders. Philadelphia, 1990.

Powers and Howley: Exercise Physiology. Brown & Benchmark, 1997.

Prentice, WE: Rehabilitation Techniques in Sports Medicine, ed. 3. WCB McGraw-Hill, 1999.

Prentice, WE: Therapeutic Modalities in Sports Medicine, ed. 4. WCB McGraw-Hill, 1999.

Prentice and Draper: Therapeutic Modalities for Allied Health Professions. 1998.

Preparticipation Physical Examination, ed. 2. Prepared by the following medical associations: AAFP, AAP, AMSSM, AOASM, McGraw-Hill.

Rachlin, ES: Myofascial Pain and Fibromyalgia: Trigger Point Management. Mosby, 1994.

Rankin, JM, and Ingersoll, C: Athletic Training Management: Concepts & Application. Mosby, 1995.

Ray, R: Case Studies in Athletic Training. Human Kinetics, 1995.

Ray, R: Case Studies in Athletic Training Administration. Human Kinetics, 1995.

Ray, RR: Management Strategies in Athletic Training. Human Kinetics, 1994.

Ray and Wiese-Bjornstal: Counseling in Sports Medicine. Human Kinetics, 1999.

Rothstein, JM, Roy, SH, and Wolf, SL: The Rehabilitation Specialist's Handbook. FA Davis, Philadelphia, 1991.

Roy and Irvin: Sports Medicine: Prevention, Evaluation, Management and Rehabilitation. Prentice Hall, 1983.

Snider, RK: Essentials of Musculoskeletal Care. American Academy of Orthopaedic Surgeons, 1997.

Spence, AP: Basic Human Anatomy. Benjamin/Cummings, 1990.

Starkey, C.: Therapeutic Modalities, ed. 2. FA Davis, Philadelphia, 1999.

Starkey and Ryan: Evaluation of Orthopaedic & Athletic Injuries, FA Davis, Philadelphia, 1996.

Street, S, and Runkle, D: Athletic Protective Equipment: Care, Selection and Fitting. McGraw-Hill, 2000.

Study Guide for Management of Bloodborne Pathogens by Athletic Trainers. Human Kinetics, 1997.

Sullivan and Grana: The Pediatric Athlete. American Academy of Orthopedic Surgeons, 1990.

Thomas, J: Drug, Athletes & Physical Performance. Plenum Publishing, New York, 1990.

Thomas, CL: Taber's Cyclopedic Medical Dictionary, ed. 17. FA Davis, Philadelphia, 1993.

Thomas and Nelson: Research Methods in Physical Activity, ed. 2. Human Kinetics, 1990.

Thompson and Floyd: Manual of Structural Kinesiology, ed. 12. Mosby, 1994.

Tippett and Voight: Functional Progression for Sports Rehabilitation. Human Kinetics, 1995.

Torg, J: Athletic Injuries to the Head, Neck & Face, ed. 2. CV Mosby, St. Louis, 1991.

Torg, J, Vegso, J, and Torg, E: Rehabilitation of Athletic Injuries, ed. 2. CV Mosby, St. Louis, 1991.

Torg, J, Vegso, J, and Torg, E: Rehabilitation of Athletic Injuries: An Atlas of Therapeutic Exercise. Year Book Medical Publishers, Inc, 1987.

Torg and Shephard: Current Therapy in Sports Medicine. Mosby, 1995.

Turner, Sizer, Whitney, and Wilks: Life Choices: Health Concepts & Strategies, ed. 2. West Publishing Co., 1993.

Valmass: Clinical Biomechanics of the Lower Extremity. Mosby, 1996.

Voss, Ionta, and Myers: Proprioceptive Neuromuscular Facilitation: Patterns and Techniques, ed. 3. Harper and Row, 1985.

Wadler and Hamline: Drugs & Athlete. FA Davis, Philadelphia, 1989.

Wardlaw and Insel: Perspectives in Nutrition. Mosby Yearbook, 1993.

Wilmore, JH, and Costill, DL: Physiology of Sport & Exercise. Human Kinetics, 1994.

Williams: Introduction to Nutrition & Fitness & Sport, ed. 4. Benchmark & Brown, 1995.

Wright and Whitehill: The Comprehensive Manual of Taping and Wrapping Techniques. U of Alabama, Cramer Products Inc, 1991.

Zachazewski, JE, Magee, DJ, and Quillen, WS: Athletic Injuries & Rehabilitation. WB Saunders, Philadelphia, 1996.

Ziegler, T: Management of Bloodborne Infections in Sport: A Practical Guide for Sports Healthcare Providers and Coaches. Human Kinetics, 1997.